Constipation

Natural Plan to Cure Your Constipation Forever

(The Easiest Way to Eliminate Constipation and Cleanse Your Body)

Richard Fields

I0146615

Published By **Regina Loviusher**

Richard Fields

Constipation: Natural Plan to Cure Your Constipation Forever (The Easiest Way to Eliminate Constipation and Cleanse Your Body)

ISBN 978-1-77485-771-7

Legal & Disclaimer

The information contained in this ebook is not designed to replace or take the place of any form of medicine or professional medical advice. The information in this ebook has been provided for educational & entertainment purposes only.

The information contained in this book has been compiled from sources deemed reliable, and it is accurate to the best of the Author's knowledge; however, the Author cannot guarantee its accuracy and validity and cannot be held liable for any errors or omissions. Changes are periodically made to this book. You must consult your doctor or get professional medical advice before using any of the suggested remedies, techniques, or information in this book.

Upon using the information contained in this book, you agree to hold harmless the Author from and against any damages,

TABLE OF CONTENTS

Introduction

We are grateful that you have selected this book as your guide for how to manage your constipation. For certain people, constipation might appear to be an everyday and simple problem to resolve but, in reality it can cause more serious digestive problems and issues in the future, if it is not addressed and treated properly.

I would also like to be awed by the fact that you have completed the first step on your journey to becoming healthier. This book should be your guide. What everyone needs to know is that you can't be completely and fully well if you are struggling with your stool movement.

This book we'll discuss everything you must learn about constipation. We will explore what causes constipation, the indicators and the signs of it, as well as the root causes that cause it as well as the various treatment options along with the variety of preventative strategies.

If you're looking to be free of constipation, then I can assist you in achieving it. My role will be to guide you through. We'll work together.

After you read this book, you'll learn valuable knowledge that can be used to aid you in battling constipation, so you can maintain a healthy and more regular functioning digestive system.

Like what I said earlier It's the first step.

Always remember that you're not alone and that anything is possible provided you have enough patience, determination , and determination to alter some of your unhealthy lifestyle and dietary habits which are not serving you.

You are able to be free of CONSTIPATION. I will explain the book with you how you can achieve this.

Thank you again, I hope you have fun!

Chapter 1: Understanding Digestion

In this section, I'm going to talk about the way that the digestive system functions as a basic guide.

First of all, the food we eat and how we digest food plays an important impact on our overall health. Being plagued by chronic digestive issues could be anything from constant diarrhea, to heartburn to gas. It's not something we'd want to see on our adversaries!

Digestion is a complex process in which both chemicals and biological organisms break down substances that are introduced into our bodies. In the digestive tract, it is divided in two parts that are the digestive tract (the stomach, mouth duodenum, esophagus and stomach) along with the lower tract (small and large small and large intestine). Food is broken down by the upper tract, and then moves via the lower tract concluding in the large intestinal tract as waste material.

In the mouth, salivary glands produce enzymes that aid in breaking the food before it's swallowed. Together with the crushing motions of your teeth and a bite of salad is transformed into a mushy paste, called bolus. It is the foundation that begins its journey to all of the digestive tract.

Many people are suffering from digestive problems because of this first step, namely not chewing their food correctly. Each step of the process is crucial.

As food passes through the esophagus, your body goes through a sophisticated process. Highly effective digestive chemical (hydrochloric acid as well as pepsin) as well as billions of bacteria working to your benefit, will determine if what's going down is beneficial or harmful. If you consume something that causes an adverse reaction at this point the body will then have to take the necessary steps to eliminate it (and we're all familiar with is involved).

The stomach and small intestine are assisted by the pancreas, the liver and gallblader that all execute complex tasks, ranging from purifying the blood, releasing the bile, and breaking down carbohydrates, fats, and proteins which our stomachs are ineffective at handling without assistance.

The enzymes in these organs are combined with the various sections of the small intestinal tract (a 20-foot coil) which include the duodenum, jejunum, and the ileum. The duodenum continues to breakdown food items, while jejunum and the ileum are responsible in helping the body absorb the nutrients. Within the small intestinal billions of microbes help in the process of breaking down.

The remainder of the waste is transported through the large intestine, or colon. In the beginning, it's in liquid form before the colon is able to divide the liquids. The stool is kept in the upper region in the large intestine, known as the sigmoid colon. This is before contractions take place that push it into the rectum prior to being eliminated. In these phases diarrhea is as the body responds in response to the existence of pathogens, not separating the liquids when it attempts to eliminate it. Constipation, on the other hand, occurs when too much fluid is eliminated.

Health and Digestion

Know that 35% of your immune system is housed in your digestive system. This is due to the fact that the health of the building blocks of your body (less than every a dozen years your body has recycles all of its cells and is an "new individual"!) And your present health is heavily dependent from the purity of the food that enters the sacred spaces within your body. The digestive system has to defend itself against all kinds of foreign harmful elements, and even dangerous but commonly-used bacteria like Ecoli. The digestion immune system is constantly at work.

It is also the reason issues with your immune system can affect the digestive tract. Stress and overload have been proven to weaken immune systems. It frequently occurs in conjunction with digestive issues; from heartburn to getting more ill from small amounts of pathogens found in your food.

The health that your digestive tract (and consequently your immune system and the entire body) is largely dependent on the healthy bacteria present within your body. In reality, the number of microbes in your body is greater than the number of the cells you have around 10 trillion. This is equivalent to around four pounds of your body mass , which is merely bacteria! They also outnumber the cells that make up your are made of (approx.. 10-to- 1)[11.

The colony of bacterial colonies is known as microflora. In addition, they are directly affected by the foods you consume. Certain foods can promote the right kinds of microflora. Likewise, certain foods can harm the microflora. The overall health of your digestive system is dependent on keeping these people healthy.

In the modern world , we continuously introduce substances that harm our digestion or encourage negative bacteria colonies. The foods that our bodies do not have the capacity to could be considered disease-causing agents or as foreign intruders. This is the case with artificial sweeteners as well as highly chemically laden food items with preservatives.

Another aspect that is crucial to your digestion health is your acidity of your diet. The degree of acidity or the pH of your system can influence your digestive system in general and could be one of the main causes of issues. For instance, the stomach can be extremely acidic and has an extremely low Ph however, should it become too acidic the acids may begin to consume the stomach's lining which can lead to ulcers. In contrast, if the digestion system was too alkaline and the body's enzymes could start to fail to function effectively.

In addition most people don't look at their gut health. The most effective way to restore your gut flora is by introducing the right dairy that contains acidophilus. We'll talk about this later. probiotic cleansing is one of the most effective methods to quickly relieve common digestive issues that are chronic.

Our diets are the biggest element of all. From eating food that isn't fresh, or consuming an unidentified food allergy we could be damaging the gut flora and decreasing our immune system and hindering digestion without conscious of it.

Why should you go natural?

It is possible to ask why it's best for people to "go natural" when it comes to digestive remedies. The reason is that most, if not all of the over-the-counter digestive treatments are made to treat symptoms, not solve the problem.

For example, Imodium solutions to treat diarrhea (Loperamide) make use of an ingredient that blocks the body's attempts at expulsion of an infection through the flushing of stool. The main issue with this method is the fact that the root cause stays within the body. Although it's unpleasant (and possibly dangerous if it can dehydrate you) however, what's more harmful is Ecoli bacteria that are ravaging your gut and causing inflammation in the intestines, without flushing mechanisms in place.

The most important question you should think about before you purchase the Loperamide drug is: how can bacteria be expanding so quickly within my body in the first place? Why do I experience persistent diarrhea or am I suffering from food poisoning frequently? The reason could be the absence of a the healthy glut flora or a weak immunity, or any other reasons that we'll look into more thoroughly throughout this publication.

Then, we'll offer antacid tablets. These tablets are designed to temporarily improve the digestive system's pH. They are utilized to treat heartburn symptoms gastritis, esophagitis and stomach ulcers by making the acidic environment into an alkaline one. However, after the antacid has worn off it's still an excessively acidic body! The antacid only served as an aid to a larger problem.

There are a myriad of digestive medicines that function in this manner, starting with Pepto Bismol to anti nausea medications. While these medicines are helpful in relieving symptoms but if you have persistent digestive issues it's an error to rely only on these medications.

This is the reason why digestive aids, supplements to your diet and remedies, or probiotic cures are the only solutions to fix the condition of a digestive system over the long term. The problem with using short-term solutions will be that you're leaving the main issue to go on unabated. As time passes and you get older your digestive system is bound to become worse, and you'll need more medication. You'll obviously, you'll have to shell out much more when your doctor switches your treatment to more powerful medication (with more side effects and more!).

Chapter 2: Digestive Problems Causes And Lifestyle Changes

This chapter will look at the causes of most digestive problems and what lifestyle and diet modifications you can adopt. These are the most effective first steps to take to treat digestive issues prior to moving on to the real solutions in chapter three.

Frequent Food Poisoning Symptoms

We've all experienced what it's like when your digestive system isn't working. Insanely onset gas regular visits to the bathroom or the bathroom, a sour stool (foul smell or burning sensations inconsistent) and abrupt stomach cramps, often intense vomiting or pain or even an outbreak of fever.

Many people (including this writer) have experienced issues in which the attacks happen again and repeatedly. For example, it could happen one, two or even 3 times per month. We might take everything from the fridge and then discover that we are still sick!

There are a few severe diseases must be on the lookout for. These include ulcerative colitis as well as Crohn's disease. Hypochondriacs might be surfing Google late in the late at night, sweating as we learn about the possibility of these ailments.

It's not likely that you suffer from either or both of these conditions. Most cases of persistent abdominal discomfort are caused by less severe reasons. It could be due to persistent gas that remains for weeks, days or even months after initial symptoms begin to manifest.

What's going on?

Most of the time it's an outcome of repeated exposure to microbes or pathogens. Contrary to what you've heard about the urban legend that "stomach flu" isn't a real thing, there's an thing called a "stomach virus". The flu can cause bloating or digestive problems, but they aren't a digestive-related virus. The viruses that target only those of the digestion system are uncommon, with the exception of the occasional appearance of rotoviruses or Norwalk virus. Much more common than these rare diseases are the regionalized episodes in food poisoning. For example, if an grocer sends out an assortment of lettuce that is that is infected by common culprits such as salmonella or e-coli. It's not that difficult for these pathogens for them to begin making people sick.

Another reason could be that food items in your pantry are creating a bad odor but you don't stop eating it, and reintroducing the microbes. If you're constantly feeling overwhelmed, it's the best thing you need to determine what you've been eating, and then avoid the food items for a few days. There are numerous common causes like:

- Unfresh deli meat

Do not wash your vegetables and fruits.

Food contamination - eating from a contaminated area or using a dirty dish sponge

- Inflammation of an undiagnosed allergy to food

I would suggest that you cut off the normal supply of food items from your pantry. Go into your local organic grocery store to purchase Greek yogurt and probiotic shakes as well as other acidepholus-rich or positive bacterial strains. Reduce your intake of foods that are difficult to digest for a few days, and concentrate on fruit and yogurt with your yogurt. You can also try one of the cleansing methods that I'll discuss in the future.

When you experience food poisoning One of the most common mistakes is not allowing the body to heal from episodes of sickness. It's crucial to allow your body enough time to rid itself of the pathogens and rebuild the healthy gut flora. If you don't, after a bout in which you've had food poisoning you're likely to suffer from:

Bloating and chronic gas

There are many possible reasons that you are constipated. All people experience gas as a consequence of the process of fermentation of food through your digestive system yeast, flora, and so on. The gas that we generate is actually a mix of nitrogen, oxygen, methane, hydrogen, as well as carbon dioxide. [2]

Gas and gas-like symptoms is usually the result of an unbalanced digestive system. The most common cause I've observed is that, yet again, there's an imbalance in the flora of the stomach, and food isn't getting taken in the correct way.

It's not uncommon for people who are recovering from food poisoning to suffer persistent bloating for a period of two or three months following. It happens when a body doesn't receive the right time and nutrition to heal from the harm caused by the illness.

One illustration is when a person has even a minor illness like salmonella or e-coli poisoning but once the symptoms subside, the person is back to eating heavy meals like deep-fried meats, simple carbs (white pasta, bread) or anything else that is heavy on the body and difficult to digest.

The digestive system's immune system has been at work to rid itself of pathogens. Consuming food that is difficult to digest following any disease (especially one that is gastrointestinal) is sending the system into hyper-drive. Normally , food that is easy to digest is suddenly very difficult for the body digest.

Furthermore, gas typically is a result of other food components. You're likely to experience some gas whenever certain foods are consumed like (traditionally) beans. The reason for this is that beans are a type of leafy carbohydrate, which is difficult to digest by the body. Other legumes could cause gas, too.

Chronic gas can be a result of inability to detect lactose intolerance. Lactaid supplements can be purchased at any drugstore, and may help to compensate the body's inability process lactose from dairy. If you're experiencing gas-related issues that are a issue, you should consider speaking to an expert doctor and finding out whether you're lactose intolerance or not.

If you're experiencing gas I'd recommend removing all processed foods or fast-food items from your diet as soon as you can. Your health and digestive health are contingent upon the health of the food you're eating. The cleanliness of fast food establishments are at best questionable. Also, food products that contain chemicals could be harmful in the long term.

Certain behavior patterns can be linked to gas. Stress and shouting (or getting into fights with people of all kinds) or an inability to exercise can result in digestive problems with a myriad of causes. But, everything that affects your metabolism of the body and its interconnected health may influence digestion as well as mental health!

Indigestion and Heartburn

As high as 20 percent of population is affected by gastroesophageal reflex disorder, as per research of the National Institutes for Health[3[3. Most people deal with this disorder at some time or another, particularly when the body gets older.

Common signs include Acid reflux (burning sensation and the release of stomach acid in the throat) painless sensations within stomach, sensations of being full, gastric cramps and mild ulcerative symptoms.

Pharma companies milk indigestion ailments for everything they're worth. The over-the-counter and prescription treatments are popular and can be costly. In actual fact, Americans spend billions of dollars each year on these items.

One of the main reasons why the reason that indigestion is so widespread is due to lifestyle issues. It's not wise to spend money on alternative treatments before you first try to solve these issues by altering your lifestyle.

Based on the Mayo Clinic, the following causes of indigestion could be: [44

Food overindulgence and eating too fast.

Consumption of excessive amounts of fat-rich (deep deep) food items, greasy and oily dishes and foods that are very spicy.

Excessive coffee (lots of caffeine).

- Excessive alcohol.

Carbonated beverages that are excessively carbonated (soda).

- Stress, anxiety, anger.

Prescription medication and antibiotics.

- Smoking

Cut down on one of these causes before you move on to other remedies.

Regarding Stress

It's generally believed that mental stressors like stress result in digestive problems. There are many reasons for this. In the holistic approach that is traditional Chinese medicine It's not a good decision to consume food stressed emotionally[5[5]. According to the Chinese medicine model the most important element of healthy living is Qi (the similar life-force or vitality that fighters use to accomplish amazing feats). If your moods are skewed and your energy levels are low, it can affect the vitality of your body, and may cause harm when you instruct your body to do an action like a digestion process.

Practically speaking, from a point the perspective of practicality, stressing while eating is a sign that you are more susceptible to not chewing properly your food. This could lead to immediate problems with digestion. Additionally, stress and releases of stress-related hormone cortisol can be linked to inflammation in the body and could lead to weakened digestion processing.

The main takeaway is this, friends? Pay attention to how you feel as you dine. If you're experiencing frequent stomach indigestion, consider whether you're bringing all of your troubles to the dining table.

A few suggestions to help with the problem include not combining mealtime and work. I'm seeing more people shoveling meals into their stomachs whilst trying to work using their laptops to squeeze more hours into their day.

It's not a good idea due to a variety of reasons. You'll not only be more inattention to your eating habits, but you're more likely to choose easy-to-cook processed foods to eat. You'll also be distracted by other things rather than the food you're eating, which can put you into an anxious state while you consume your food.

Instead, make food into an experience. Avoid eating in front of your desk keyboard. Visit the dining room table for lunch as well as try thinking of something apart from deadlines and obligations.

It's the same in the home also, of course.

All Lifestyle Options to Take into Account to treat digestive problems

There are a myriad of ways your lifestyle might be impacting your health and well-being. Here are some additional things to take into consideration:

Be aware of where you eat when eating at restaurants.

Infrequent gastro-related issues could be traced to your favourite restaurant or food vendor. It is shocking to see how unsanitary the conditions in the kitchen are, even at your most loved places that you might think to be completely competent in their hygiene.

One obvious sign that you should seek out an alternative restaurant in your area is the cleanliness that the bathrooms are in. If your bathroom doesn't look sparkling and clean it is sure that the kitchen is suffering from some issues with neglect too.

Sometimes, the issue isn't so much the cleanliness of the kitchen however, but the hygiene of the company's suppliers. There's a joke that's been around for a long time in my familythat goes "Never go to the sushi restaurant situated in rural Kansas". This is a great deal of sense since for sushi to stay fresh, it is essential to take it to a spot close to the ocean. If you move further inland, it's much more difficult to get fresh ingredients for certain meals.

Certain businesses might also reduce costs by using substandard wholesalers. This is, for instance fast food outlets that attempt to satisfy large quantities of customers in a limited period of time. This causes mass processing of bizarre animal parts and replacing actual ingredients with chicken or beef flavorings (for more information on this subject I recommend the book "Food Inc").

In general, you should be careful about where you go out for meals regularly. Even if you're familiar with all the employees at your favourite café, it doesn't mean it's the most healthy location for doing your business.

Your diet is too starchy

A diet that is very starchy could cause constipation and constipation is the most common cause in stomach cramps and indigestion gas, and a myriad of other signs and symptoms.

Alongside a myriad of other health benefits your body requires fibrous matter to aid in all kinds of digestive functions. If your meals are usually associated with items such as macaroni and cheese rice, potatoes white bread, no greens at all You're at risk of a myriad of adverse consequences.

So , what can you do? Well, start eating vegetables! It's not a good idea to eat the consumption of starchy, sugary vegetables like potatoes or many other root-based vegetables (including carrots). Spinach as well as broccoli, collards greens, and Brussel sprouts are some of the kinds of food items that you must be eating.

I'm sure not everyone loves their veggies. I've heard many reasons for not eating vegetables, and many adults are still acting as if they were my five year old. If you're not fond of your green food, you can consider these suggestions:

Reduce the cooking time. A lot of people mistakenly believe that they dislike vegetables, but they are just averse to the texture that is mushy when cooked too long.

Include lemon butter. Most vegetables taste better when paired with lemon butter and salt.

Try to discover what you enjoy. You'll meet people who have never consumed certain types of asparagus previously! Don't make a judgement until you've had the chance to try it (in the actual sense, this principle applies to everything!).

Last but not least, don't not forget to include a substantial amount of kale into your diet. Anyone who has read my books will be aware that I constantly recommend incorporating this specific vegetable into the diet because it's a great source of every essential mineral and vitamin you require, possibly alleviating deficiencies that were not even aware you already had.

Your Cooking Space Is Not Hygienic

This is crucial. I've previously mentioned how a dish sponge that's dirty could make you sick. It's accurate and I've seen it occur at least once. The sponge must be removed and replaced every week at a minimum. Additionally, after using your sponge for any reason, you should squeeze out the excess water. The growth of mold and bacteria is a common problem on sponges that are moist within the pores.

Make sure your fridge is clean and empty. There are still pathogens that thrive in fridges but at a less rapid rate due to the cold environment. Although blue cheese mold can be safe if it's removed however the more serious spoilage can be identified by tiny pink dots appearing on the meat that has been spoiled. This is called salmonella (named by the person who came up with it, and who also had the same name as the color of bacterial growth). This pathogen can be extremely harmful and storing spoiled food in the same place like other food items could cause a smear of contamination. The spots of red on cheese are red cheese mold, which is more dangerous than blue mold.

Make sure that your counter is clean each when you use it, and adhere to a no-go policy on handling raw meat. If your dish has meat that was raw do not just give it a rinse, but make sure you scrub it thoroughly with dish soap that is antibacterial, and then put it in the washing machine.

Beware of cooking or cooking raw food. I've seen some naughty barbecuers put cooked chicken on a grill which isn't completely heated and then add the chicken on top of a bun in order to bake it. The bread will absorb some of the juices of the chicken but it's not likely that it'll get heated enough to kill any bacteria.

Also, don't wash raw poultry or meat with water that is near the counter, or in particular containers for food items, such as that salad bowl. It's not a good idea to wash your meat. It is better to boil it. The water's spray could carry salmonella throughout your kitchen!

Also, cook meat according to the recommended temperature for internal cooking of 166 degrees Fahrenheit. If you are making something like stuffing (prepared inside the carcass of a turkey) Be sure to ensure that the stuffing is cooked thoroughly after it's cooked. The stuffing will remain protected from the heat while taking in the raw turkey juices and can cause food poisoning.

You don't wash your hands.

There are a variety of ways to get pathogens that are on your hands such as Ecoli or salmonella, listeria and more in your daily activities. If you're prone to eye-rubbing or nail-biting this is a great way to pick up viruses such as the flu. You could also possibly expose yourself to bacteria that could lead to food poisoning.

Wash those hands!

There's no use for the Fridge

In certain cultures, the refrigerator isn't utilized more often than it is in North America. When I was a student in France I was surprised to find that French people laughing about the American habit of keeping my eggs in the refrigerator. This is an American habit that I am quite in love with.

Salmonella thrives best when it is temperatures of room temperatures. Nowadays, most of the eggs don't have the salmonella threat because chickens in farms are vaccinated against it. Studies have found that there is no differences in the levels of salmonella between separating eggs and cooling them. [6]

But, despite the findings of the study that show it's not an issue when you keep eggs in the fridge some scientists warn against egg that is kept in a room temperature as it is difficult to know exactly where the eggs come from. It's all it takes is one bad batch of eggs and you're at risk of getting sick.

I believe this is especially relevant for those who are like me and love buying organic eggs from farmer's markets. It's impossible to be too prudent in that situation and purchasing eggs that are free range eggs can increase the chance of acquiring bacteria.

(However I think it's worth it to avoid the antibiotics used in mass-farmed animals.)

Along with egg yolks, some folks even leave out milk. This seems ridiculous. Milk spoils faster when it is at temperatures of room temperature.

To be on the safer and secure side, I keep everything refrigerated even the bread, which helps it last longer. It's not as popular to spread this narcissistic American routine However, I believe that I'm sick lesser than most people.

You're not acclimatized to an Environment

Many travelers, and sometimes even going to different states within the same nation experience frequent episodes of diarrhea, indigestion or food poisoning. What's happening here?

If you've spent a long time in a certain geographic region your body is adapted to the microbes that live there which means you'll never become sick due to them. Visitors however could not be so fortunate. While we're a global society today, a lot of bugs have established long-term homes in particular areas, particularly in the food we consume.

It could take a while to acquire enough natural immunity to the new environment to fight off illness like the indigenous people have to. When you travel, make sure to have Pepto in your bag. This is especially important when you're traveling to an ethnic group with different eating practices (like traveling across the West into Asia).

Chapter 3: Your Natural Cures Guide

It's time to take a dive and find out about the tested techniques for ridding your stomach of ailment without the harmful side effects of conventional medicines. But, be aware to apply natural and herbal solutions with care. Even things that are "of the earth" could be dangerous in particular if one has an allergy or sensitivity to a particular ingredient.

Bloat/Gas

Activated Charcoal:

While it's not clear from a scientific standpoint what the benefits of charcoal are for the stomach It's been proven to aid in various gastro issues which includes gas. The kind to purchase can be described as "activated" charcoal which means that it is usually oxidized through the process of steaming. The steam creates tiny holes in the charcoal, making it porous. As we utilize charcoal to filter our water, it is a natural method of cleaning the water we drink, those pores can also trap toxins inside your body , and could be able to absorb pathogens that can cause digestive issues.

Activated charcoal is usually purchased online or at any other place supplements are readily available.

Apple Cider Vinegar:

Vinegar is yet another old and well-known remedy. First, it assists in helping maintain our pH levels through its powerful alkaline properties and it also functions in the form of an inner cleanser. If you're suffering from gas, you can add 2 tablespoons of vinegar made from apple cider into warm water in a glass.

Asafoetida:

The middle eastern herb, like leeks is an additional stomach remedy , which is typically used in food items in India, Iran, Pakistan, Afghanistan and many other nations. In particular, it is recognized as an antiflatulent and directly aids in the treatment of gas and the bloat.

For the best chance to get the herb, it is best to purchase it from a supplier. It is usually packaged and powdered. It is an excellent seasoning for various meals. If you are able to locate the herb whole (again at a reliable import grocery store) it could be the best way to instantly alleviate gas. In this type of form, it is typically consumed raw in Middle Eastern salad dishes. The aroma and taste are known to be quite difficult for those who are new to eating.

Baking soda and lemon It is a natural mixture that produces carbon dioxide, which is able to make your digestive tract more balanced during an episode of gas and is an beneficial treatment.

Fill a glass with water, and add 2 tablespoons of lemon juice, and 1 1/2 teaspoons baking soda. Stir it with a spoon and watch it begin to bubble. When the fizz has diminished take a sip of the tonic.

Fennel: Similar to asafoetida, it is a different herb that is native of the Middle East and many parts of the Mediterranean coast. It is a sour, aromatic herb utilized in numerous dishes from this part of the world. Fennel seeds can be found in numerous Italian recipes, including sausages and meats that are cured.

In addition to being a plentiful ingredient, fennel is also famous for its digestive aid and, in particular, for curing gas. Take a bite of dried seeds of fennel (with sufficient chewing). A lot of people report that following this, gas is instantly eliminated from the area where it could get stuck in the intestinal tract.

Fennel seeds can cause some adverse consequences, especially for people suffering of epilepsy. It is important to determine whether fennel is suitable for you prior to consuming any.

Ginger: This root is renowned for its digestive qualities and has been utilized to treat digestive issues for hundreds of years. When it comes to treating gas or gastric bloating, it's extremely effective. The most effective kind of ginger is, according to me, is known as Gari that is an Japanese thinly sliced salmon-pink-colored young ginger. It is typically served with the majority of meals served in Japanese restaurants , and may be pre-sliced in certain supermarkets in foreign countries.

Consume 9-10 pieces and chew deeply.

Ground Turmeric:

Based on research of scientists at University of Maryland medical center[7The spice turmeric can provide numerous benefits for digestion which include stimulating the gallbladder to produce bile.

Turmeric is generally found in powdered forms. It is then used in numerous applications and recipe ideas. You could try adding 2 tsp of it to the milk in a glass full (creating the appearance of a golden hue and also a delicious taste). Also, you can discover it in many mustards that are spicy. Mustard is also a source of health benefits too, which could aid in digestion. Try eating 2 tablespoons of mustard it's self.

Turmeric can be purchased in a variety of health food stores shops, and can be ordered on the internet.

Probiotic Cocktails: You've seen me talk about prosbiotics' importance to digestion health. But what many people aren't aware of is that there are lots of options other than yogurt that can provide an effective and quick relief to stomach gas-sufferers. Try:

- One half cup Sauerkraut

2 servings of Kimchee - 1-2 servings (Korean fermented cabbage dish). It is available at foreign grocery stores and Korean restaurant.)

3 whole pickles

1-bottle of Kefir (sour fermented milk drink)

One cup buttermilk

or 1-2 servings yogurt with probiotics.

Spearmint or Peppermint Tea (or Essence of Mint

Menthol is the active ingredient in mint, is renowned for its anti-nausea qualities. Mint-o-philes also claim that it could be an easy fix for episodes of gas or other stomach upsets.

Find a pure version of peppermint teabags. make tea by steeping it in boiling water and covered for about. 15 minutes, to make an intense cup. You can add a little sweetener (preferably honey) and take a sip.

Insomnia as well as Heartburn Natural Cures

Here are some treatments to look into for indigestion ulcers and heartburn that could be causing it.

Stress:

To not sound like an old record, but I have mentioned the causes of tension and indigestion previously. What are specific steps you can do to instantly reduce the negative feeling within your life?

In the beginning I believe that most instances stress can be removed. My brother had an infected ulcer at an extremely (unnecessarily perhaps) stress-inducing time during his lifetime. However, the majority of his anxiety could have been eased (as as the medical bills) should he had taken a few steps to unwind.

I could write a second book on stress relief. But I believe the best method to deal with stress is to address your issues, so that you don't have to fret about these issues. This could be the pile of bills that are on the table, or the tough conversation with someone you've put off.

Meditation can be beneficial however, if you've got unfinished business in your head I'm convinced that it's difficult to find the time to even contemplate.

Personally, if I have something that has to be taken care of and I've not completed it then no amount of relaxing music or other methods will help.

Find out the root of your issues to begin putting them together, and then begin knocking them out of your head! After you've finished everything and you're done, it's more easy to relax.

Then, once you're at a point where you can relax enough to let immediate stress go out of your mind, I'd advise that you begin to practice meditation. I discuss these kinds of ideas more in depth in various books.

Increase Acid Levels

This may sound odd It may sound odd, but medical professionals have found that acid reflux is usually caused by lack of acid and not due to having excessive amounts. The lower esophageal muscle tightens when acid levels drop and tightness then sends the remaining acid into the digestive tract.

The ways to increase acidity are:

The juice of 1/3rd of the lemon, squeezed into the glass of water and topped with a little sugar (a powerful lemonade)

Sea salt

- Apple cider vinegar

- A few servings of acidic fruits.

For salt, the most effective choice is the one that is not processed (Himalyan) which is likely to be the best solution for balancing your acid levels. This is due to the fact that chloride is utilized by your body to create (hydro)chloric acid that is the chemical you consume in digestion to break down food. The salt replenishes this chemical in its uncooked form.

Try spreading it on some veggies, such as steaming cabbage.

If you are considering fruit, consider it as a last resort since acidic fruits are often difficult to digest and can cause the symptoms to worsen.

Also, be aware that vinegar and lemons have an unorthodox property in that they're both acidic and alkaline (I'll go into more detail about this in a moment). Numerous health experts agree that it's best to keep your body alkaline. Fortunately, combating an imbalance in pH isn't the same in the same way as acidifying it and these food items will raise your alkalinity levels overall.

Ginger:

As mentioned before, ginger works digestive miracles. Alongside taking a bite of the pink Japanese ginger I'd recommend purchasing some the tea made from ginger.

If you purchase the tea from a retail store beware of powdered or green "herbal" tea. It is best to purchase sliced or chopped fresh ginger which can be steeped in the same way in the same way as a regular teabag.

A lot of health food stores sell Ginger in the form of. Let the tea steep for 20 minutesbefore you put the pot in the refrigerator to keep it warm whenever you notice symptoms of indigestion.

Stop the Medications:

OK. Certain medications can cause heartburn and stomach indigestion and the patients do not even realize that they are suffering. These side effects could be more severe if they are coupled with an unhealthy diet as well as if the medicine was consumed without adequate food items in your stomach.

Certain drugs that can cause indigestion due to a reaction are:

* Antidepressants
* Anti anxiety
* Blood pressure
* Antibiotics

Don't necessarily stop taking your medication. Instead, speak to your physician about the indigestion issues you are experiencing and establish an appropriate timeframe for when you'll be able to quit taking the medications.

In our day and age I am aware of many patients who take anti-anxiety and anti-depressant medications and never complete their requirement for these drugs. The concept behind these medications is that patients take them the duration they have a problem. After that, with psychiatric therapy patients don't need to take them any longer.

However, they keep using the same medication for years and years with all the unpleasant negative side effects that accompany these drugs.

If you experience digestive issues or other problems as a result of these medications, consider consulting with your physician to develop a plan of action so that you do not have to continue taking them for a long time.

Alkalinity

As acid can increase your acid levels, it's ALSO feasible to manage reflux using alkalinity. This is due to the fact that alkaline properties will neutralize acid within the stomach (although it might not stop the underlying cause for acid reflux).

There are a variety of methods of getting a good dose of alkalinity

* Mustard

Like other treatments, a teaspoon of Dijon mustard can be a great alkaline boost.

* Peppers

A majority of peppers are acidic in their nature. While spicy peppers could harm the gastrointestinal tract, mild yellow ones are good (like those we consume on hot dogs or hoagies). Take a good portion with crackers.

* Apple Cider Vinegar

Another time with vinegar! It's possible that you're somewhat confused, since vinegar was advertised as an acidic remedy isn't it?

As I've mentioned before in the past, despite the fact that vinegar can be acidic in nature, it actually does have an alkaline impact in our body! Do not ask me to clarify the chemical explanations that are behind this, since I'm way out of my league. The fact is that vinegar has both acidic as well as the curative power of alkaline. That's all we have to be aware of.

* Alkaline vegetables

Certain fruits and vegetables are quite alkaline in the natural world. This includes celery Apricots, carrots and spinach and radishes, cauliflower and some dried prune-like fruits, like raisins. Start incorporating alkaline food items in your diet by cooking portions at every meal. Note when it starts to relieve the symptoms of indigestion.

The Holistic Energy Cures:

Many believe that our bodies are encapsulated with energy patterns that superimpose themselves over them. Certain emotional conditions can affect the chakras of our bodies, and this can cause a variety of symptoms like stomach acid and heartburn.

The chakra that is associated with digestion is known as Manipura Chakra[8] that is situated in the spine, and the point of activation is in the navel. In accordance with Yogic tradition the energy flowing through this region is the reason for feeling of self-confidence and confidence.

If this energy is disturbed but not fully restored, feelings of indigestion and lethargy could begin to manifest.

Take a moment to think about this, whenever you've been feeling "off the ball" have you noticed how it was followed by fatigue and fatigue? Let's say that a romantic partner has triggered you. In the following day, you could be feeling depleted of energy and not have any interest in getting up.

The best way to rekindle this Mampura Chakra is to alter your routine to keep your energy levels under control. According to holistic experts, in order to maintain this chakra's balance, you should be organised and finish tasks without fear. Therefore, if you've got twelve tasks to finish, but you're not doing switching to the mode of high efficiency.

If you start to feel confident about your capabilities, and your self-esteem increases and you feel more confident, the Mampura Chakra will be reinvigorated and maybe your digestive issues will disappear.

From a skeptical perspective I believe these practices can reduce stress as well as other chemicals which cause tension and hypertension which can be linked to ulcers. If you think it's an energy thing and not old methods will help.

Natural Diarrhea Cures

Diarrrhea may be due to food poisoning or pathogens or due to your diet when your body is lacking healthy gut bacteria. In the previous chapter, I discussed in detail getting good gut bacteria back to your system. This can be accomplished by adding foods such as yogurt with live cultures and Sauerkraut in your diet.

There isn't a quick solution for chronic diarrhea. The over-the-counter medications address symptoms, but do not address the root cause. The antibiotics could require an extended period of dosing to eradicate the bacteria that is of concern.

There are a few brands and supplements that are believed to aid in the speedy curing of diarrhea and to help keep you in good health until the potential dangers disappear.

Lactic Acid Yeast Wafers

I've heard lots of positive things concerning these delicious wafers. Like other fermented foods the wafers can help promote the development of beneficial bacteria. They're quite concentrated and some have reported that they saw diarrhea-related symptoms disappear within the first day of having one of these wafers.

I'm not able to find a source for yeast wafers. However, I believe it can be purchased at a specialist retailer. However, the yeast itself is available on the internet in supplement form and will likely produce similar effects.

Pectin

For a short-term treatment for diarrhea, it's essential to introduce plenty of pectin. It's a fiber that absorbs excess fluid. Since your body uses fluids to flush your bowels, pectin may slow this process.

The following food items are good sources for pectin

* Carrots
* Applesauce and apples
* Apricots
* Bananas
* Tomatoes
* Potatoes

One of the best sources of pectin is carrot, which is a good source, containing 0.576 grams of pectin per large carrot[9].

Pectin is also used in a variety of foods that are synthetically in order to provide gelling effects. Examples include jellos as well as custards and other desserts. But, I'm not certain how effective the synthetic pectin options are in helping combat diarrhea.

One method to treat diarrhea right away is to consume an adequate amount of both carrots and rice along with a banana or two as a side. A healthy high-starch mix such as this, that is loaded with pectin, is a good option.

Slippery Elm

The slippery elm an eminent tree found in North America with rough, long branches[10[10, 11]. Its bark is its medicinal portion, and has a long tradition of therapeutic uses. Particularly the slippery elm tree can be utilized to treat digestive issues.

One of the advantages on the bark of it is the fact that it covers the digestive tract, which in turn reduces inflammation. Certain doctors recommend the supplement to help to treat inflammatory conditions that include autoimmune issues. The digestive tract, such as inflammation of your bowels, may be a cause for your diarrhea.

It can be bought in powdered form in the health store or on the internet.

High-Fide

It seems counterintuitive it is that fiber which is thought of as a cure for constipation could aid in preventing diarrhea. In reality, fiber assists in general stool control. Increase your intake of fiber by a few grams per every day. You can do this by eating a few portions of green vegetables and bran muffins.

Staying Hydrated

It's essential to stay hydrated if you have persistent diarrhea. This is the reason why diarrhea can become a fatal disease, with diarrhea causing pathogens such as cholera which cause many thousands of to million of deaths each year across the globe. In reality, dehydration due to diarrhea is typically the cause of death for serious illnesses such as ebola, and treatment for these illnesses focuses on water and replenishment.

Soups made from chicken are great for electrolytes. One of the most nutritious dishes you can consume is chicken broth that has been mixed with one glass of instant, or boiling rice. This will replenish your water and also help to transport the nutrients as well as smother the excess fluids.

The health food stores in your area could also carry natural "Gatoraid" type drinks that contain electrolytes drinks, free of harmful dyes. Make sure to have these drinks on hand during an outbreak of diarrhea. If you're constantly going for a bathroom break, you can rest sure that you're getting dehydrated .

Understanding the Root of Your Diarrhea

Different remedies need to be tailored to specific factors. Diarrrhea can be either an osmotic or infectious condition. Causes that are infectious will be addressed within a short period of time, and can be caused by an infection caused by a virus, bacteria, or even a protozoa or parasite. In the second case it could be as simple as being diagnosed with an amoebic disease due to contaminated water and then having an infectious worm growing in your digestive tract.

Infectious diarrhea is extremely hazardous if you do not see an expert doctor and use appropriate medication. This is the reason why chronic diarrhea must be handled by a professional immediately. The reason that so many people suffer from diarrhea in the developing nations is due to the lack of medical treatment. If you're able to access medical treatment, don't allow it to go.

In the same way the mere occurrence of a few days of symptoms is likely not enough to cause concern It will most likely go away.

Osmotic diarrhea could be caused by other causes that include gut flora imbalances that we spoke about previously. It can also be caused by treatments, immune disorders, such as Crohn's disease or drug regimens such as cancer patients who undergo chemotherapy.

In these instances, treatment options are only able to treat the symptoms, since the root cause might be difficult to address.

Constipation

Constipation may occur without reason or rhyme, but it's typically caused by changes in diet or moving to a different place. Sometimes, constipation is also a result of diarrhea, which can lead to a prolonged period of digestive issues.

Constipation is often simple to treat with natural remedies. There are numerous kinds of food items and supplements that can be used as natural laxatives, without having recourse to the recourse to a chemical.

Olive Oil:

The first quick fix for constipation recommended by a naturopath. Simply take a teaspoon of olive oil combined with lemon juice to make it more digestible. It is recommended to consume the dosage in the morning prior to eating breakfast. Olive oil is known to stimulate the colon.

Olive oil is superior to the castor oil that is simple awful. But, according to some reports, the effectiveness of castor oil can be greater when you're in a hurry.

A Hearty Meal:

Perhaps the first thing to do once you've stopped needing"go "go" is introduce the fiber. A lot of people experience constipation after eating simple carbohydrates (white pasta, breads and other breads) along with other starches. When you consume these foods there's nothing leafy to aid in the process of removing the waste. The starchy foods then bind the food waste and block your colon. Fibers aren't digested like different substances, and therefore they help keep the stool from becoming a mess.

The following food items must be considered for inclusion:

-- Bran Muffins (Can help relieve constipation)

Prunes, figs raisins, apricots, pears fresh or dried.

Breads made from whole grain

Legumes of all kinds.

High fiber cereals

- Leafy vegetables (asparagus, spinach, etc).

Mix it with probiotic yogurt. Reduce consumption of starchy food items. Avoid foods that are difficult to digest like fried or fried meat and.

Prunes are among the antiquated remedies to treat constipation. The active ingredient in them is dihydroxyphenylisatin which can help in maintaining healthy colon health.

Consider a Diuretic Natural

A diuretic that a lot of people have heard of is coffee. Consume a single medium cup of coffee with a fibrous snack such as a bran muffin.

Take note that caffeine may have the opposite (constipating) impact, too. This is the reason it's not advised to drink more than a cup of coffee. Actually, it could be the cause of the frequent constipation you experience. If you're addicted to coffee, try to cut it out to a minimum, as well as different sources of caffeine and observe if there's an improvement.

Other natural diuretics include lemon and pineapple. However, their effects might not be as fast as coffee. It is still possible to try the pineapple juice or lemon-water, and check out what happens.

Magnesium

According to some experts[11According to some specialists[11 (see the footer) magnesium deficiency can be the cause for a myriad of symptoms, which range from heart problems, and constipation.

If you're experiencing frequent constipation and your physician isn't sure of the reason, it could be that you aren't getting sufficient magnesium intake in your daily diet.

Magnesium is a mineral which is found naturally in several food items. This includes:

- Leafy vegetable--again, asparagus, spinach, kale broccoli, and various greens are rich in tiny quantities of magnesium.

Seaweed is known for its levels of magnesium.

- A variety of seeds and nuts. Particularly squash, pumpkin as well sunflower seeds.

Another good source of magnesium is the mackerel fish. A portion of this fish has an average of 97 mg, which is 24 percent of your daily requirement.

Due to the comparatively low supply of magnesiumin the world, it's not a surprise that the majority of people don't manage to meet their daily intake of this mineral.

Certain people opt for magnesium supplements Also. However I prefer getting it from the raw sources, which are in fruits and nuts.

Flaxseeds

Another high-fibrious food that is also a good source of omega 3 essential fats.

Additionally the fibrous nature of it can aid in the health of your colon.

Flaxseeds can be found in abundance at grocery stores that sell health foods. They can be eaten for a snack or even add them to your yogurt with probiotics.

Blackstrap Molasses

Another home remedy that is of some reputation. Molasses is sweet and rich in calories. However, it can act like an occasional laxative. If you do not would like to experience the edge of a sugar-induced high I would suggest limiting the amount you consume.

Diet and exercise

Another reason why many people experience constipation is due to their life in a sedentary state. Your body must be active to ensure that functions like colonic movements can be carried out quickly.

Sitting for long time periods can interfere with these processes.

If you work at an office job or have a lot of time at a desk it is important to take regular break for exercise. Jog, walk, or do a few quick exercises such as squats and sit-ups.

Many people also purchase mats for their workplaces. Spread one on the floor every now and then take a breaks to exercise each day. If you are seated in one spot too long could cause more severe problems than constipation!

Chapter 4: Restoring Your Digestive Immune System

The majority of digestive problems may be due to suffering from an "unclean gut". The primary defense against external contaminants can be your intestinal flora which is the smallest part of the intestine. They is the bacteria which capture the invaders, then absorb and kill them. pathogens.

If the membranous layer of beneficial bacteria gets damaged by the same invading bacteria that a healthy person can easily ward off may make you in a state of digestive discomfort for months, weeks, or even for years.

As time passes, it is possible that our defense against bacterial infections becomes weak. Then, we don't have the time to correct it.

Common Reasons Why Your immune system or gut flora is Broken

Antibiotics

The main cause of a bacterial colony that is unhealthy is the continued or previous use of antibiotics. Antibiotics work in the end as an effective weapon against bacteria-related infections. They kill large quantities of pathogenic bacteria in addition to all your beneficial microbes.

It's not uncommon to encounter digestive problems after a dose of powerful antibiotics.

A Period of Physical Stress that is Intense

Your flora in your gut isn't all positive. There's an entire plethora of microbes that are different, and the kind of colony you're a part of is contingent on a variety of aspects, such as what you consume and your general immunity.

Your immune system some moment was functioning at a high rate and weakened because of it this could give the opportunist bacteria an opportunity to grow. If your digestive tract is deficient of the beneficial critters and they're less likely to help you.

Rebuilding your immune system as well as creating a cleansing routine that is probiotic can restore your balance of your flora.

Unhealthy Digestive Organs

Your pancreas and gallbladder as well as your stomach, kidneys , and the liver all play a role in the health of your digestion. Constantly exposed to toxins or stress could cause digestive issues at best, but deadly illnesses such as cancer at the extremes.

The following are the possible ways that your digestive organs could be affected:

- Smoking

- Excessive alcohol

A diet devoid of nutrients (constant pizza, pasta white bread, etc.)

- Constant exposure to chemicals

A large amount of use of pharmaceutical drugs over a long time

Your digestive organs are affected by what is entering your body. The kidneys and the liver for example are directly involved in the process and elimination of substances. It is possible to overload these organs, which is the reason those who drink heavily end up developing liver cirrhosis.

If these organs the well-being of your entire digestive tract will be affected.

Persistent yeast infection

The growth of yeast can occur in your body due to an immune system that is compromised, and then cause further harm to the health of your digestive system. One of the places where yeast is identified to grow is on the digestive tube within the tube itself. A healthy digestive tube serves as the primary defence against harmful bacteria. If yeast begins to overtake healthy bacteria in this space that could lead to that there are many uninvited guests.

It's not that yeast is harmful, however. In fact, it is a part of the collection of beneficial microbes. The only problem is if yeast starts to "rule the dominion" within your digestive tract.

Autoimmune Disorders

There isn't conclusive proof that priobiotics can have any effect on the autoimmune diseases such as celiac disease, Crohn's disease or inflamed bowel conditions. If you experience GI troubles persist regardless of the cleansing process the bowel, it may be an indication that there is an autoimmune issue and you should seek the advice of your physician.

Parasitic Infections

It's difficult to believe, however, a lot of us suffer from parasitic illnesses (often worms) that can lead to chronic digestive issues. In the coming days, I will explain how to manage these issues. There is no need to be worried!

We'll now look at some options to cleanse yourself and improving your digestive health.

A Probiotic Basic Cleanse

A cleanse is essentially the strict control of the food you consume. There are many benefits to using cleanses, ranging from weight loss, to identifying any food allergies to strengthening the immune system.

Probiotic cleansing is intended to provide your body with plenty acidophilus in its natural form. Yogurt is in my opinion the best method to transfer the bacteria. Therefore, yogurts must be supplemented by non-diary cultures for those who are lactose-intolerant.

Finding and purchasing Probiotics

A priobiotic can be identified in the form of "Live active culture" printed on its label. It is important to pay attention to the amount of organisms when that number is stated in addition to information about storage to ensure the organism is active. Sometimes, you'll see an item that recommends cooling at room temperature instead of refrigeration.

Be cautious when purchasing products that are treated commercially. The heat treatment of yogurts implies that a lot of these bacteria could end up dying. Specific processing methods must be employed by businesses that want to ensure that live cultures remain persisting inside their goods. If you purchase on the internet, the probiotics need to be delivered while kept in refrigerators.

Be wary of packaging that states the quantity of bacteria "at the time of production" because it will be considerably less when the packaging process is completed.

The amount of live organisms that are present ought to be about 1 billion for an efficient probiotic supplement.

I am still skeptical about acidophilus chewable supplements that are dry and chewable. Because we're being dealing with living things, I can't think they could survive being stored in a dry place for a whole month.

Identifying the Bacteria

There are four major cultures that the majority of products support. To get a great cleansing, it is recommended to reenergize your body using the four "heavy weights".

Lactobacillus acidophilus: The common bacteria that you will find a lot of discussion about as a nutrient-rich component of many dairy products. Acidophilus aids in all sorts of digestive functions and has its primary function of converting lactose into lactose acid.

Lactobacillus bulgaricus: A different important gut microbe that is identical in its function and structure to acidophilus. It is also present in dairy products, including yogurt and cheese.

If you purchase yogurt products, be sure the bacteria is included.

Streptococcus thermophiles is a bacterium that processes and extracts nutrients from various food items you consume. it can also be found in yogurts. It is not associated with the Strep bacteria that cause the strep throat.

Bifidobacteria is a bacterium family that regulates digestion processes, and a deficiency of this bacteria can result in digestive health problems.

The products

You can purchase your bacteria in supplement form or purchase live bacteria at your local grocery retailer.

When you purchase a supplement it is essential to ensure that it is refrigerated prior to transport, and has large amounts of many bacteria which includes the four I mentioned.

After lots of research and comparing, the brand I'm with is Number One

Nutrition. they offer their product as a capsule. It's quite affordable compared to some other brands that cost higher prices and for much less, and has proven to be efficient for me.

For dairy, I recommend going to the store (I like Whole Foods) and looking through the selection of active cultures. I'd suggest:

2 active culture shakes
1 box of at least 12 yogurts with active cultures in small amounts
Optional: Active culture cheese
Be aware of the label and search for any asterisks in the active organisms. If it states "at the time of production" return it and it's probably less useful than regular yogurt.

I have used Activia and have found it to be effective. However, many people prefer off-brands and local brands. The reason for this is that the simpler the manufacturing process, and the faster it gets from the manufacturing facility to store shelves the less likely that the current culture has been disrupted.

The Yogurt or Dairy Probiotic Cleanse

A good cleanse lasts, in my opinion, two days. Some doctors recommend to continue a cleanse for 5-7 days in order to get the maximum impact. In certain situations it might be beneficial. However, it is dependent on the kind of cleanse you'd like to undertake. If you are taking a probiotic infusion I believe that you can see outcomes in a shorter amount of time, provided that you keep the probiotics as a routine component of your diet following the.

I completed my first (2 days) cleanse similar to this during the midst of terrible GI symptoms that persisted for throughout the entire week, caused me to be miserable. The symptoms disappeared quickly and I've not been plagued by even slight amounts of gas and bloating, or diarrhea, or any other stomach ache for nearly two year since I did my initial cleanse. I'll repeat this routine at least once per year.

Breakfast 2 servings of healthy yogurt, with granola that is high in fiber.

Lunch 2 portions of yogurt with active culture as well as a small amount of active cheese and Whole grain bread.

Dinner 2 servings of active yogurt from culture, with a with a side of digestible vegetables and fruits (I recommend cucumber).

In both days: sip in your yogurt smoothie.

If you started at 8 am the previous Monday morning, you may end it at 8 am on Wednesday.

During the cleanse, drink huge quantities of liquids (water). Avoid drinking any other fluid other than water. This includes sweet fruit juices or alcohol-based drinks.

Once the cleanse is finished Reintroduce normal, more nutritious foods.

Fermentation Cleanse

Yogurt is a kind of food that is fermented, however there are other options to pick from if you want to stay away from dairy or simply want to mix things up a bit. All in all, incorporating a variety of fermented foods in your diet could help alleviate various digestive issues.

My opinion is that there's one minor drawback when choosing dairy and non-yogurt products. That's because companies are less focused on cultivating certain live bacteria. A portion of sauerkraut or kimchee can be technically made from living organisms. However, absent a specialist retailer, it's usually difficult to know the quantity of living organisms in the product.

If , for instance, it's a brand name of the common Hotdog Sauerkraut, the quantity of beneficial bacteria may not be sufficient even.

Therefore, you should shop for specialty items, and be sure to look at "live the culture" printed on labels, regardless of the type of product.

It is possible to mix it up with a variety of food items like live pickles, miso that is not pasteurized or fermented beverages such as kombucha and the fermented ("German type") mustards.

For bases, go for dark Rye. There are also processed meats that people love however I don't have any prior experience in this field.

A few of these foods could be a little more difficult to digest in comparison to a pure yogurt cleanse. Therefore, I suggest the first cleanse if are experiencing GI upset.

Concentrate on eating only the mixtures of these fermented foods and drink lots of water. The cleanse will be completed within a few days, and then reintroduce regular foods.

Gallbladder Cleanse

A few doctors suggest cleansing the gallbladder in order to improve the digestive system. The function of the gallbladder is to store bile created by the liver. It will release it as needed. It is essential for breaking down fats. Foods that are heavy may be difficult on your body if the gallbladder is not performing well. Of course the gallbladder isn't the most vital of organs, since if it's removed , your body shifts to storing bile in the ducts.

This is a cleanse originally listed at DrDavidWilliams.com[12]. He recommends:

Organic cider and apple juice.

Disodium phosphate capsules

- Citrus fruits

Unrefined olive oil

- Lemon juice

Every morning, drink huge quantities in organic ciders.

In the afternoon, eat as usual. At around 3 pm take 3 disodiumphosphate capsules and 8 ounces of water. Repeat the process with 3 capsules with the same amount of water three hours later.

Make sure to limit your dinners to more juices, and concentrate on citrus and grapefruit juices. Then, before bed take a cup of oil that is unrefined, followed by a small amount of grapefruit juice or half a cup warm unrefined olive oil , paired with 1/2 cup lemon juice. Personally, I'd suggest the former since it's more enjoyable.

Be prepared for "unusual" dark stool, clumps which form "marbles" that are which are softened by the increased use of gallbladders. The doctor. Williams also warns you might be experiencing uncomfortableness in your quadrant surrounding the gallbladder. However, take it easy about it.

He recommends that you continue this cleansing for five full days.

For Parasite Infections, Cleanses and Cleaning

One thing to think about is the uncomfortable idea that there are parasites in your body. As per the World Health Organization, 3.5 billion people suffer from parasites. The parasites are a common occurrence in nearly all mammals, with humans included.

Most parasites are known as helminthes--primitive worms that have evolved alongside us.

A parasite infection may theoretically be a long-term digestive issue that refuses to be going away. It can be difficult for doctors to recognize that the issue is caused by parasites therefore, if you're experiencing a recurring digestive issue that is not explained particularly after returning from a trip to a country that is developing it is advisable to consider the possibility of a parasite.

Below are the top commonly encountered parasites:

Roundworms/Whipworms: There is a reason to thoroughly clean all fresh produce since even an "organic and premium" fertilizer may still have roundworm eggs. They are found in the intestines as small worms with threads. The symptoms that are visible are not common.

-- Ascarid: The ascarid roundworm is one the biggest parasites. Imagine a huge earthworm-like creature that is in your intestines , and produces numerous babies. It's among the most frequent parasite-related diseases (over one billion people are affected) and, as terrifying as it sounds, the majority of infections don't cause symptoms and are not harmful (some researchers believe it's because humans have lived with them for many millions of years, and our bodies have become adjusted to them, and they could even play as a way to boost our immune systems). But, if they're not controlled, infections can pose a risk especially for children.

Tapeworms: The most frequent symptom of a tapworm is the ability to regulate weight. It may sound as if it's a positive thing however, your shrewd digestive pet is also hindering your ability to take in nutrients. Tapeworms can be found on raw or badly cooked beef pork, fish and other meats. A single tapeworm may be as long as 12 feet or more, and is composed of a tiny main body, and infinite egg sacs.

Pinworms: Tiny white worms. They are a part of your colon and escape in the night through your rectum , where they lay eggs on your anus. They come back into their colonies. The primary symptom is itching. Pinworms can be extremely infectious and the majority of us get them at some point or at a different time. It is likely that they are not related to digestion. issue since they can be detected when they are present (persistent Itching in the rectal) and can be treated with an over-the-counter medication for pinworms from any pharmacy.

Parasites used to scare me However, the positive side is that these pests are simple to eliminate and virtually harmless and the majority of parasite infections not causing any symptoms for the duration of their existence. That's right there are much more serious issues to be concerned about.

There are additional risky parasites to be aware of in the event of acquiring. For example, uncooked or raw pork could carry trichinosis, an invasive worm that can infiltrate the brain, often killing the patient.

The dangerous parasites are more rare than they are, but it's a helpful reminder to prepare your food.

How to deal with Parasites

I've never witnessed such a large amount of hypochondria in my life before studying forums on natural health about parasites. The majority of people believe they have parasites , they start seeing them everywhere they travel. One woman's post said she was even able to mistake the phlegm as parasites! They also talk about their battle with worms over time and how even after multiple cleaning treatments, the parasites persist. Unfortunately, this hypochondria was designed by companies who want to market their anti-parasite supplements. What these snake-oil firms do not want to advertise is the majority parasites are killed immediately after you take an anti-helminth drug. This treatment is not costly and is likely to be less prone to side effects than an anti-parasite cleansing, which may be difficult to take.

The website could provide you with the symptoms of parasites that are common to everyone or may be a myriad of other things. You'll then see an image of how the ugly little creatures appear like, and you'll be freaked out and click on the "buy" click.

However, this doesn't mean that all the natural solutions to parasites are not effective. They work however, and if you're not opposed to using the medication when you suspect that you're suffering from an ailment, it may be worth giving it a shot.

To cleanse your body Here are some basic.

Garlic: It is designed to weaken parasites. It's recommended to take 3-4 gel capsules per day in between meals. Expect to get plenty of garlic breath, and possibly nausea.

Wormwood, Black Walnut, Thyme and Cloves: Taken as supplemental forms. Make sure you read the directionscarefully, avoid overdoing it, and make sure you purchase from a reputable supplier (not the first item you see when you search on Google). These supplements are intended to convince the worms that they will be more enjoyable in the drainpipe, rather than in the intestinal tract.

Probiotics can strengthen your body's defenses and reduce the possibility of worms re-entering your body. Take yogurt and probiotic supplements.

Light meals and liquid food It is recommended to take a week to incorporate an effective juice cleanse in addition to the other supplements mentioned above. Liquid meals such as kale and apple smoothies can be able to help. Make sure you drink plenty of water as well.

There could be other health benefits of undergoing such a diet in addition. It's definitely worth taking a look. But remember that doctors will not recommend this as the only defence if you suffer from an infection that is confirmed, because although mama's tapeworm is gone and many of her sisters have been eliminated it is possible that there are plenty of eggs to be found. This is why , ultimately, taking a pill is the most effective solution to rid yourself of all trace.

Eliminating Consumption of Hard to Digest Foods

In the end, cleansing and treatments aside, you'll never be completely free of digestive issues if you do not take the time to remove food items which can cause digestive problems. It's important to learn what your body's capabilities are at digesting and what isn't. For instance, some people have a good tolerance for spicy foods, while eating lots of jalapenos might be making you sick.

If you are unsure you are unsure, avoid all of them:

The Spicy: as I mentioned, take out the hot peppers for a few minutes. One of the most common side effects can be acid reflux.

Sodas: high in acidity as well as High fructose corn syrup artificial ingredients such as food coloring and other chemicals. The body doesn't know how to handle soda after it has entered.

Caffeine: Caffeine relaxes the esophageal muscle, which could result in acid reflux and digestion. Coffee, however, is an effective natural diuretic.

Saturated Fat: Cooking bacon, pork and sausages can result in lots of saturated fat, which is accompanied by tough to process, heavy fat molecules. If you experience frequent digestive problems, then you must completely eliminate any source of saturated fat at least for a brief period. Saturated fats can cause diarrhea, as your body strains to eliminate it.

Drinking alcohol, particularly hard alcohol, can cause inflammation. It's not surprising that after having a night of drinking it is possible to experience digestive problems in the morning.

Desserts: Consuming a lot of sweets will certainly cause digestive imbalances. Be mindful of moderation when eating any kind of white flour pastry or pie dishes or cakes.

All Fast Food: Get rid of all food items! There are many reasons to. For example, McDonalds and similar companies frequently use a form made of wood pulp called cellulose used as the "filler'. It is not nutritionally beneficial, however it is difficult for your body to break down, leading to gas and gastric bloating. This is only one of many reasons to avoid these establishments.

Chapter 5: The Causes Of Constipation

Constipation is caused when the colon being stuffed with stool for too long. The colon is able to absorb excessive amounts of water from stool, making it tough and dry. It is making it more difficult for the muscles that make up the rectum expel the body.

Factors that could cause constipation include:

A diet which there is a lack of fiber - which is what one can find in plant food items. Fiber makes stool more soft and move effortlessly within the colon.

Adults over the age of 65 generally don't have enough fiber in their diets due to the fact that they don't consume enough of:

* Food doesn't taste as good as it used to, so people have less food to eat;

* They don't feel hungry as often because of the reduced amount of activity.

* They might not be able to cook, or

They may have issues with swallowing or chewing due to their teeth being lost, false teeth, and sometimes due to arthritis or nerve damage.

Food items that are simple to prepare or purchase like fast foods or prepared food, can thus be their first choice for food items. These products are usually high in fiber.

Physical inactivity - Constipation is often a result of an accident or illness in which a person is restricted to bed and is unable to exercise. Inactivity is thought as one of the main reasons constipation is commonplace in older people.

The use of medicines is often linked to constipation. This can include:

* antacids which contain calcium and aluminum;

* anticonvulsants that reduce the abnormal electrical activity of the brain to avoid seizures;

* antispasmodics to prevent the muscle from contracting suddenly;

* Calcium channel blockers (CCB) (or calcium channel antagonists)used to treat high blood pressure and heart disease.

* diuretics that aid the kidneys eliminate blood-borne fluids;

* iron supplements;

* drugs to help treat Parkinson's disease (a nerve disease) because they affect nerves that are located in the colon wall.

* some antidepressants

* OTC laxatives which loosen stool and improve the amount of bowel movements.

While some people may experience relief from using laxatives, they generally have to increase their dosage over time since the body is reliant on laxatives in order to get an bowel movement. Laxatives that are used excessively can hinder the capacity for the colon to contract and cause constipation to become worse.

The long-term use of laxatives may result in damage to muscles, nerves, and other tissues that line the large intestine.

* pain medication, particularly the narcotics.

* None of the OTC pain relief medications (Advil, Tylenol, Excedrin etc.) as well as OTC antihistamines (Benadryl, Zyrtec, Claritin) could cause constipation.

* Opioid pain relief medications (Vicodin Percocet, Vicodin, Oxycontin) can cause constipation. However, they can only be purchased by prescription. Continuous use of painkillers with dihydrocodeine or codeine may cause constipation. The generic names of this medications include:

* Codeine
* Buprenorphine
* Fentanyl
* Hydrocodone
* Hydromorphone
* Meperidine
* Methadone
* Morphine sulfate
* Oxycodone
* Oxymorphone
* Tramadol

Life's changes can be a catalyst for changes in everyday routines - pregnancy or age, as well as travel can cause constipation.

* During pregnancy, hormonal changes can result in constipation. Also, the uterus could squeeze the intestine, which hinders the flow of food particles through your abdominal.

* Aging can impede regular bowel movements as a result there is a gradual loss in nerves that stimulate the

muscles of the colon, leading to a decrease in the activity of the colon.

* Traveling can alter a person's eating habits and routine, which is why they aren't eating normally or frequently.

Doing nothing to avoid having the urge to bowel move - People who don't bother to use the restroom might end up not having an bowel movement. There are people who have "toilet fear" and are unable to resist the need to have a bowel tidal due to the fact that they do not desire to use the toilet outside their house, particularly bathrooms in public areas, or because they think they are too busy to sit down for the short amount of time that it takes to use the bathroom.

Disorders of metabolism and neurology can slow down the speed of food passing through the digestive tract.

The most common neurological disorders are:

* Spinal cord injuries that could cause compression in the digestive tract.

* Parkinson's disease

Diabetic-related neuropathy that can result in constipation or diarrhea.

* Strokes

O Metabolic disorders can include:

* Diabetes that blocks the mechanisms that our body utilizes to obtain the energy it needs from its food.

Hypothyroidism, that causes the body to produce insufficient thyroid hormone. This results in many of the organs to become less efficient.

Gastro-intestinal(GI) tract problems - can cause a narrowing of the colon and rectum. The causes of these problems are:

* Adhesions are bands of tissue that join the loops in intestines , blocking the flow of blood.

* Diverticulitis, an illness that develops when small pouches, also known as sacs, grow that push past weak points

in the colon wall , preventing the flow in food particles through intestinal. They may also cause severe discomfort.

* Polyps are growing in flat or raised forms on the surface of your colon. Sometimes, a large polyp can hinder or block your bowel. This can lead to diarrhea, constipation and abdominal pain as well as vomiting.

* Tumors is a swelling of an area of the body without inflammation, triggered by an abnormal increase in tissue. This can be benign or malignant.

* Celiac disease , an intolerance to gluten, an amino acid present in rye, wheat, and barley. Gluten affects the intestinal lining and blocks the intake of nutritional substances.

Functional GI Disorders - are that result from changes in how the GI tract functions. Constipation caused by functional disorders can result from issues with muscle activity in the colon or the anus, which hinders stool movement.

The condition is usually experienced by those who have been suffering from symptoms of constipation , such as struggling to get a constipation, lumpy, hard stool, or feeling like the stool is not fully eliminated after a bowel movement and for at least six months. It is common for them to take laxatives in order to aid them.

Chronic dehydration: Water accounts for more than half of the body's mass the form of interstitial, intracellular cerebrospinal fluids, cerebrospinal fluids, and blood. These fluids join the various organs and systems of the body into an efficient organism, which allows to perform many of the vital body functions.

When the body becomes accustomed to dehydration over time, people become less sensitive to water deprivation and aren't drinking when they're asked to. This could result in a sturdier stool that is more difficult to pass and can cause irritation and weakening of the colon's walls which can lead to diverticuli. If there is a shortage of supply of water within your body, it is likely that the colon may respond by limiting the excessive water loss through stool.

The colon's muscles will contract to remove all water from the stool, and then absorb water into circulation. However, this water reabsorbed is considered to be a waste, and has to pass by the liver as well as kidneys for filtration. Organs that are affected be stressed because they are performing more work than they normally do. The end result is that chronic dehydration could cause liver damage or kidney failure. This can then trigger an endless cycle of dehydration as the kidneys begin to fail - yet they nonetheless, they must work in removing the toxins that are in the water.

Stress is the most frequent reason for constipation. Stress is caused by emotional stress caused by worry, anxiety or sadness, especially when it is prolonged. The most prominent area of the body that can "feel" stresses is your digestive tract and in particular the colon. The colon's muscles tend to tighten rather than having their normal peristalsis that allows waste to flow through the colon to be eliminated. Stress triggers the sympathetic nerve system (the known as "fight and flight" reaction). Certain body types react to stress by reducing the movements that the stool moves. When stressed individuals may consume unhealthy food, reduce their exercise routines engage in and consume less water and are all frequent causes of constipation.

Caffeine can affect the digestive system since it acts as a diuretic. It also speeds up the digestion process, and also stimulates the colon. Caffeine can either cause or prevent constipation.

A diuretic, caffeine is a diuretic that affects both kidneys and the colon. In the beginning it triggers any liquid consumed to move through the body faster than it would normally. The kidneys take extra liquid from blood process it, and eliminate it as urine. So when caffeine is introduced into the system, it triggers an increase in urination, which means less water is able to reach the colon.

The colon is the organ that moves solid waste via peristalsis in the small intestine into the rectum. This requires the colon to absorb some excess fluid, as otherwise, the stool will always tend towards diarrhea. Caffeine, however, may cause the colon to absorb excess fluid in a hurry, resulting in the body becoming dehydrated.

Being Out Of Alignment

There is a reason for this, the fact that your bones are out of alignment could result in constipation. If your bones, particularly those that are located in your spinal column not in alignment, it could affect the flow of nerves. For instance, some bones that are not aligned in the lower back could cause difficulty in having an effective elimination. You may be amazed by how an easy adjustment from an experienced chiropractor can help you get back on track.

Modern-day Plumbing

This won't be popular with the majority of people, however our modern plumbing is a contributing factor to constipation. Being at a 90-degree angle is not helpful in eliminating the number two. If you're sitting at the right angles above the toilet, you'll end up benting the rectum, which makes it harder to stop the bowels with a forceful movement.

The most natural method to rid yourself of the problem is to squat that every camper who has been around for a while recognizes by "A Bear Squat In The Woods". If you're in one of the world's first nations and haven't traveled to S.E. Asia then you're probably not familiar with the toilets on the dirt. What I refer to as"the "Thai toilet" is one you stand on or rather squat onto instead of sitting. It's odd if you've not been there before but it's actually quite logical. The toilet design is designed to put your body into the ideal position for elimination , exactly as it was intended to be.

When I was traveling through S.E. Asia I lost an enormous amount of weight and weight around the middle. I believe this was due to a better elimination process all around. You might not want to install an "Thai toilet" inside your home because your family and friends will probably think you're nuts and that could make selling the home quite a difficult task.

If you're looking to reap the health benefits associated with"Thai Toilet "Thai Toilet" there are a variety of exercises and postures for your body. They're to be covered in the coming chapters.

Consequences of Constipation During Chronic Periods

If untreated, chronic constipation can have a negative impact on your life quality as well as cause stress and reduce your overall sense of wellbeing. People who are constipated for a long time:

The symptoms include depression, mood fluctuations, and unusual fatigue

* Bad breath • Bad breath and body odor;

• Loss of appetite.

More grave consequences (from the least serious to most) are:

Internal hemorrhoids, External hemorrhoids or any combination of both. The most common term used of hemorrhoids would be "piles".

Internal hemorrhoids typically do not cause pain, but they can be extremely bleeding.

External hemorrhoids can cause itching, pain and extreme sensitivities.

* Anal fissures are a crack within the skin around the anus. They result from an abrasion and stretching to the anus caused by hard stool. Common signs include:

There is itching, pain, and small amounts red blood in the stool or on the underwear.

Infections that result in an abscessthat must be surgically drained.

* Rectal prolapse is when the rectum gets too stretched because of the continuous accumulation of large quantities in stool. It will be unable to contract back to its previous size once

stool is removed. The tissue that is loose then extends through the anus and forms tiny, pink lump or bubble. Rectal prolapse is a surgical issue. Rectal prolapse is a common symptom. include:

The leakage may be small of mucus or stool;

A sensation of defecation that is incomplete;

o Pain, itching or bleeding.

Fecal impaction refers to an accumulation of stool that is hardened and is unable to pass in a normal manner.

o Impacted stool may require manual removal. The health professional will insert his hands in the rectum and break the stool into pieces. It is a painful procedure however it is quite easy.

O Medications, like stool softeners, or supplements for fiber, can also be employed. Additionally mineral oil enemas could be used to soften impaction of the feces, but they're not very effective in the removal of large impacts.

Sometimes, fecal impaction could cause megacolon (a expansion that of the colon) or lead to an entire obstruction. In this situation, urgent surgical intervention may be needed to clear the obstruction.

"Lazy bowel syndrome" (LBS) is when the bowels fail to function correctly, and they require laxatives in order to maintain regular stool movements. Regular use of laxatives may result in dependence that can worsen LBS and could result in other complications like injury to the intestinal tract as well as insufficient absorption of nutrients and vitamins.

* Bowel perforation happens when the solid fecal matter penetrates through the intestine's wall and flows in the abdomen cavity. It is a common cause

of severe infections due to the fact that the waste products of the body are brought into direct contact with vital organs. The serious disease (called peritonitis) resulted from this discharge of waste products from the abdominal cavity could be fatal if not addressed immediately.

* In the elderly constipation is a chronic condition that takes the large intestine away from its mucosal membrane, which is thin and leads to polyps and flat lesions which can lead to colon cancer.

Helping to relieve constipation

The treatment of chronic constipation requires an integrated, holistic approach to lifestyle:

Maintain a regular routine that includes going to the toilet at the same time every morning. Set this as your morning "habit" because the colonic motor activity is at its highest at this point.

Be aware of your body's movements: Peristalsis, the movements that cause bowel movements or come and go. If you ignore the urge to go, it is a sign that the opportunity could be missed. If stool is left in the bowel for too long, it becomes more difficult and harder to eliminate because more water is absorbed. The desire to flush is higher after eating and you should be attentive to the body's signals.

Relax: Since stress can hinder relaxation of the entire body, including the bowels, a certain type of relaxation routine is advised. In addition, taking enough time and the privacy you desire will allow you to unwind when you go to the bathroom, and also allow for an easier passage of stool.

Drink more fluids to maintain a healthy lifestyle: Drink plenty of fluids. It is recommended to consume at minimum 1 glass of fluid (preferably water) per 10 kilograms of body weight every day, and even more during hot weather as well as when you exercise.

Incorporate more bulk into your diet: Dietary fiber as well as bulk fiber laxatives, such as methylcellulose or psyllium combined together with lots of fluids could help alleviate constipation that is chronic.

Consume light meals on a regular basis Make sure that you consume food minimum 3-4 hours prior to the time you go to sleep. Regular meals do not just reduce constipation risk They also boost the rate of metabolism and help to lose weight.

Get medical advice regarding medication: Laxatives and medications can ease constipation however, they should be used cautiously and only for short intervals of time. Numerous medications, supplements, or herbal remedies may cause constipation.

Perform regular physical exercises

The general movement of the body can help in constipation elimination, but certain movements are more efficient than others. Certain exercises and movements help to align the digestive track and eliminate track to ensure more thorough elimination. If you're able to have more complete as well as more thorough elimination you'll see that you'll be healthier virtually in a matter of minutes while your overall energy level will rise!

Simple Home Remedies to Help Relieve the discomfort
Home remedies typically comprise of a mix of vegetables and fruits seeds, fiber, seeds and oils.
Fruits and vegetables
* Raisins contain a lot of fiber and work as natural laxatives.
* Guavas contain soft pulp with soluble fiber and insoluble fiber inside the seeds. They also aid with production of

mucus in the anus, and also in the peristalsis.

* Lemon juice dilute in warm water is acidic and aids to increase digestion.

* Figs, whether dried or ripe, are stuffed with fiber, and are an excellent natural laxative. The use of a whole fruit in this purpose is superior in comparison to syrups which are sold in stores.

* Oranges are rich in fiber content. Consuming oranges two times a day can be a great way to relieve constipation.

* Spinach is a plant that can cleanse, restore and rejuvenate in the intestinal tract. A mixture of Spinach juice and the same amount of water two times a day is the most effective way to get rid of even the most challenging cases of constipation.

Seeds
* Flaxseeds are renowned for their high levels of fiber. Fiber is an essential

ingredient to your daily diet. It helps to reduce hypertension combat diabetes, combat heart disease, combat overweight and lower the risk of developing cancer.

* Seed mixtures made of flax seeds, sunflower seeds, sesame seeds, and almonds ground into an extremely fine powder could assist in relieving constipation.

* Chia Seeds are one of my top choices for keeping me regular. They're not just filled with Omega-3s, they also bulk up quickly and aid in the cleansing of the intestines.

Fiber

A fantastic solution for constipation at home is to consume fiber ranging from 20 and 35 grams daily. Fiber can also be a useful remedy since the majority of people have items made of fiber at home. Supplements made of fiber are also available.

The issue when taking fiber as a home solution (both natural and supplementation) can be that it could cause more constipation in the absence of ample water. Fiber requires fluids in order to help in peristalsis.

Good sources of fiber include:

The Bran grain and the other grains are are found in cereals whole wheat, seeded or whole wheat breads, brown rice, and other breads;

*Vegetables like asparagus Brussels the sprouts as well as carrots as well as collard greens and kale are fantastic for washing you up!

The fresh fruits like Apple provide the highest amount of fiber and are dried or fresh figs. If you're trying to be healthy and regular, you should eat at five figs a day!

Chapter 6: Remedies To Utilize With Caution

* Castor oil has been utilized throughout history as a treatment for constipation. It also contains ingredients that eliminate intestinal worms. It is not recommended to take it in the evening due to its fast effects. Another disadvantage of this treatment for constipation is that it is a bit bitter and is much easier to consume when chilled and blended with a sweetener, such as orange juice. The oil of castor is regarded as to be safe, however it could cause overdoses if consumed in large quantities.

* Fish Oil is a rich source of Omega-3 fatty acids, which are believed to play a role in digestion . It can also help in the treatment of Crohn's Disease and ulcerative colitis. This includes constipation. Fish oil consumed in your diet through eating cold-water fish,

such as mackerel, salmon, halibut and sardines, herring, tuna or through supplements that contain omega-3 fatty acids, is a good source of these fat acids.

* Aloe Vera Juice

Aloe is ideal for getting things moving naturally, as the Aloin present in ale Vera aids in breaking down food that is affected and sucked up in the digestive tract. Aloe Vera Juice is a great alternative to laxatives that your body may be dependent on. The possible side effects are diarrhoea, which can happen when taken in excessive amounts quantities. One or two glasses per day of aloe vera juice can help, without causing any undesirable adverse negative effects.

* Coconut Oil

Unrefined Coconut oil isn't just the perfect supplement to healthy diet, but also has many various other applications for health and wellness too. If you suffer from constipation, try taking just 1 Tablespoon of coconut oil in the mouth or mix it with your morning cup of coffee. Once you've become accustomed to the unrefined, raw coconut oil, gradually increase the amount to 4 tablespoons daily.

* Vitamin-C

Vitamin C can be very beneficial for loosening the colon, so make sure you are aware of that. It is a good idea to take Vitamin-C to bring the flow back however if you take too much, you could end up having a swollen stool. It is important to play around on this issue. It is recommended to begin with the recommended dosage in the bottle of Vitamin-C supplements and then adjust it to your requirements.

Fish oil supplements must be used with caution since the high amount of omega-3 fatty acids may increase the risk of bleeding. People who are easily bruised or suffer from bleeding disorders must be cautious when taking this method. Another side effect that is negative can be that the fish oil may cause gas or bloating and, in certain cases, cause diarrhea.

Kombucha

Kombucha can be described as a fermented drink which has been used to promote better health throughout the world. Similar to many traditional remedies that have emerged of the woodwork lately, Kombucha has become more industrialized and is now available to purchase it at the grocery supermarket, while before you were required the ability to create it yourself. The health Benefits of Kombucha are improved immunity, better elimination and detoxification. Other benefits that can be observed from Kombucha areless joint pain, increased vitality and feeling of well-being.

Kombucha's components comprise sugar, tea, and the starter culture. The purchase of Kombucha from the market is easy, but making it yourself is enjoyable and also less expensive.

Herbal therapy is among of the most ancient forms of treatment for constipation and many cultures across the world have relied on herbs to treat constipation for a long time. The constipation treatment is usually divided into two types: stimulant and bulk-forming laxatives.

The stimulant herbs that can help constipation include senna Cascara segrada and aloe. However, stimulant-based laxatives, especially aloe, can trigger cramping. Therefore, senna would be the better option. Alongside the adverse effects, herbal treatments for constipation could be incompatible with medicines and other supplements. Always consult with a certified health professional prior to taking any herb.

The most commonly used bulk-forming herbal laxatives comprise both plants and sees, including flaxseed, fenugreek, and barley. If you choose to use flaxseed for the first time, bear to keep in mind that the flaxseed oil may not be identical to oil extracted from the actual flaxseeds. They can be purchased as whole or as crushed seeds. Flaxseed oil isn't designed to be a remedy for constipation and shouldn't be utilized in this way.

Foods To Avoid

Foods to avoid

To avoid and relieve constipation, it's essential that healthy eating habits are established. Certain foods can trigger or worsen constipation. These foods must be avoid, including:

Gluten or wheat

Today, wheat is far from the grain that was once the staple of our predecessors. There are many people who have developed sensitivities to any ingredient in it as a result of the processing that is overly geared towards wheat products and other wheat-based ones. The process itself has altered the grain's molecular structure and may cause gas, constipation, and bloating. Adhesive substances like glue are made from gluten and wheat products. In case you do not wish for anything to become stuck in your intestines , then it's time to eliminate the wheat!

Dairy Products

Be cautious when you are doing too much with dairy products. Except for fermented foods like kefir or raw milk cheeses, the majority of dairy products are extremely processed and are very difficult to digest. If you have to consume dairy products, limit your consumption to small portions and try your best to limit yourself to high-quality goat cheeses, raw milk cheese , or fermented beverages like Kefir. Yogurt is beneficial in the long run, as long as you choose yogurts that have low sugar levels.

Caffeinated Beverages

Consuming caffeinated drinks throughout the day could cause digestive problems. Because caffeine is diuretic in effect, you're getting rid of fluids and water that must be kept in the flow of fluids in your digestive tract. If you must drink coffee, make sure to stop drinking after 12 pm and consume water throughout the day. If you can do that one small thing you could discover that staying consistent is not difficult.

Foods that are processed

This includes everything that is produced in a factory or prepared in oils that are produced in factories. The most likely culprits include items like baked goods, cookies snacks, chips, snack foods, and more.

Red Meat

If dairy can be a problem for your intestines, then red meat can be even more difficult. Reduce your consumption of red meat to once or twice per week and choose a high-quality red meat. If you stick to organic meats that aren't contaminated with antibiotics and hormones, you'll be able to see that any negative effects such as feeling constipated and bloated are less of a concern. Another reason to eat organically-harvested meats is that they are more natural in flavor, as well as vitamins and minerals.

Frozen Dinners

Most frozen meals are lacking in nutritious fiber. In addition that the majority of them are extremely processed, which can make people constipated.

Bananas

This is a fascinating one. While I was an nanny, a long time back, the mother of the child I cared for informed me that if the child was experiencing diarrhea, I needed to provide him with bananas to help make him constipated. A reliable source advised that unripe bananas could cause constipation, while ripe bananas are able to help ease constipation. It is possible to experiment and see which one works best for you.

Diuretics

If the constipation you're experiencing is prevalent, it's a good likelihood that you're dehydrated, also. You should stop drinking drinks that help to eliminate fluids from your body. You require enough fluids like water to ensure that things are moving around in your body. Drinking too much beverages or coffees can cause things stuck inside your body, items that you don't want stuck.

If you're worried about feeling overweight, constipation can increase the severity of your problem. Believe me, I've been there and have experience in this area. Avoid or reduce the intake of the intake of things that have a high amount of carbonation, sugar, and caffeine. In addition, your digestion tract be grateful, but your kidneys and liver as well.

Exercise
Aerobic exercises like running, walking, swimming cycling, dancing, or walking are among the most effective exercises for relieving constipation issues. Aerobic exercise increases the flow of blood towards the organs as well as the gastrointestinal tract, which assists in peristalsis as well as generating more digestive enzymes. Both of these help in the passage of waste from the digestive tract. Engaging in a vigorous lifestyle and doing three hours of exercise per week could help keep people healthy.

Yoga is also a great way in relieving constipation. Yoga practitioners recommend specific postures that help stimulate the digestive tract and bring the energy flowing into it. The twisting and bending moves in yoga can help move stagnant materials in the body.

Exercise can also be beneficial for stress management because it increases neurons to produce neurohormones, such as serotonin, norepinephrine, and norepinep which are connected with better mental function, a higher mood and increased learning.

The most effective exercises to treat constipation include:

* Walking

Walking is a great way to alleviate constipation via stimulating the peristalsis pump. Ideally, you'll want to walk for at least 20-30 minutes each day. According to one source that you should take 10,000 steps every day to maintain the best health. 10,000 steps per day is five miles, or 8.04672 kilometers. How long would it be?

It's entirely up to you. One suggestion I give to many is to begin parking your car farther away from the store's entrance before you are shopping. You'll not only gain more walking time, but, when you return to your vehicle, you'll be in a position to get out of the parking quicker!

* Yoga

Yoga offers many postures that , if you practice them regularly can assist you in saying goodbye to constipation permanently. Below are examples of poses which can help to shape the track of elimination and increase the digestion process and eliminate. Certain of these postures or positions could be more difficult for those who have knee problems. I will offer two categories of poses to relieve constipation. The first group is for those with no knee issues. The second group will be designed specifically designed for people who have knee problems.

Yoga for People With Knees that are Healthy:
*Garland poses (Malasana)

* Chair pose (Utakasana)

* Extended Child's Pose (Utthita Balasana)

* Cobbler's Pose (Baddha Konasana)

Yoga For Sensitive Knees:
* Relieving Pose to Wind (Pavanamuktasana)

* Plow Pose (Halasana)

" Half Lord Of Fishes (Arha Matsyendrasana)

* Corpse Pose (Savasana)

Breath Of Fire

Breath Of Fire is a deeply beneficial breath, which if you practice it regularly can be used to heal and restore many weak systems of the mind and body. When it comes to constipation it aids in exercising the diaphragm as well as to build your digestion. Avoid it if are pregnant or experiencing menstrual cramps.

You can sit on the floor in a crossed-legs or on your knees or sitting in a chair in case you have knees that are sensitive. All breathing goes in and out via the nostrils. Hands are at ease. It is possible to place one hand on your diaphragm and make sure you're lifting the diaphragm during the inhale, and then relax the diaphragm during the exhale.

Chapter 7: Constipation Explained

Constipation is a common condition that affects anyone of any stage of life. When one is constipated the process of removing stool is often a struggle. People who are constipated may also experience less frequent bowel movements as than those who do not suffer from constipation.

This problem will differ from one person to the next. It's not usually a major issue however this doesn't mean that there isn't any attention required to take care of it. Similar to what I previously mentioned within this article, a healthy individual must have regular stool movements to eliminate the waste the body does not require. Furthermore the time that constipation is chronic, it could cause not just discomfort and pain as well as a decrease in quality of life and health issues also.

You might be asking yourself this question: How can I know if my constipated?

What you must remember is the fact that frequency bowel movements can differ from one person to the next. The normal routine for certain individuals may not be normal for others and the reverse is true. For instance, it's typical for me to experience every day bowel movements. What do you feel? Do you see my point?

In general, not having stool movements for three days straight can be considered to be long already. After this time, the feces might become more challenging to get rid of due to the fact that they've hardened.

For reference it is considered constipated when you have been experiencing at least two of these for at least three months.

Stools can be hard for over 25 percent of the time.

It is not possible to pass your stool for at a rate of more than 25% the time.

It is difficult to pass stool for more than 25 percent of the time.

A bowel movement or less every week

CAUSES OF CONSTIPATION

There are many reasons for constipation. In this article we'll discuss a few of the most commonly reported causes. The below list to determine if you're susceptible to developing constipation, or not. This list could also aid you change unhealthy habits you have.

• Insufficient intake of drinking water

You might have heard who advise you to consume at eight glasses of water every day. This is accurate. However, it is important be aware that an individual might require more or less than this amount according to the health condition and overall state of his the health. For instance the case of someone who does regular exercise, he or she might require more fluids. In contrast doctors might restrict your water intake in the event that you've suffered from heart problems.

This is why you must know yourself well as you have needs. If you're people who are active You may require more water as compared to people who aren't as active. In simple terms your water requirements depend on your health and your current health.

* Insufficient fiber content in the diet
Another common reason for constipation. Fiber can help to increase the volume of your stool to facilitate digesting and eliminating. Furthermore fiber is also known as a way to help move food items through into the digestive tract. Apart from aiding in fighting constipation, fiber can also help combat various ailments in the digestive system, like acid reflux or Inflammatory Bowel Syndrome.

In the next chapters, we'll be discussing fiber further, and the best foods that are rich in fiber.

* A sudden change in diet or routine
Certain people might experience constipation because of sudden changes in routine or diet. It is a common occurrence for travelers. Due to this, we suffer from what is

known as constipation caused by travel.

For some, this could be due to the "safe-toilet condition". What we need to know is that the body is generally relaxed during toileting.

If we go away from our homes, like when traveling, we could be uncomfortable. This is why it can be difficult to move stool.

* Inactivity levels that are not high and exercising

Yes, you got it right! The lack of exercise could result in constipation. If you don't get sufficient exercise routine, then the length of time food items will travel through your intestines will take longer. As a result, more water is taken in since the duration of the food is increased. This can make your stools less palatable.

As per experts' advice, it's suggested to train for 20-30 minutes per each day. Exercise is essential not only to help prevent constipation but also to maintain your weight and overall health in check.

* Stress

You might be wondering how constipation can be caused by stress. The reason for this is really quite easy. When you're stressed out this could affect and affect the relaxation of your body and digestive system. Most people are unable to effectively empty their bowels because they are in a hurry or aren't relaxed and stressed out.

The key here is to avoid rushing your bowel movements and slow down as much as you can.

* Pregnancy

Women who are pregnant are more susceptible to constipation due to the hormonal changes their bodies go through. Additionally when they are in the final stage of pregnant period, the uterus could restrict certain parts of the intestines, slowing the normal movement of food.

* Aging

As we get older, we could expect that our metabolism will slow down. As a result, there is also a lower activity in the intestines that could increase the risk of constipation.

* Dairy products

Some people who are lactose intolerant might experience constipation following consumption of dairy products.

* Excessive use of laxatives

If we become addicted to laxatives the body is likely to not notice the effects of it until we boost the dosage. In the future, after we cease taking laxatives there is a greater chance of becoming constipated.

OTHER potential causes

* Different neurological diseases like Parkinson's disease, multiple Sclerosis

* Medicines such as antidepressants and antacids

* Colon Cancer

REMEMBER:

Constipation is not thought of as a medical condition. It is a sign that is caused by a variety of reasons including those mentioned below.

SIGNS and SYMPTOMS OF CONSTIPATION

Similar to what I said earlier, when you experience constipation, your frequency of your bowel movements may be less frequent than in normal. It could also be extremely difficult to get stool out. Due to this, the most typical indication of constipation is slowing of bowel movements. In addition the straining that occurs when you pass out stool is another indication.

Here's a list of the symptoms and signs of constipation:
* Less frequent bowel movement
* Constantly straining while handing out stool
* Stool is dry, hard and lumpy
* Stool is unusually small or large.
* Feeling overwhelmed
* Feeling sick
The stomach is aching.
* Stomach cramps
* A loss of appetite
For children, here are a few additional signs and symptoms of constipation (aside from those mentioned above)
• Lack of energy
* Irritable
* Unhappy

* Stain that is foul-smelling
* Feeling uncomfortable

Note ADVICE: The frequency of bowel movements can differ from one individual to the next.

Warning Sign of Constitution

In this chapter, we'll examine some of the warning signs be aware of when you're constipated. This is especially important for those suffering from chronic constipation.

Constipation can be a common issue for some individuals, however if you notice any of the symptoms listed on the list below you should consult your physician immediately.

Abdominal pain

x Swelling of the abdomen area

Black or dark stool (It could refer to it's blood that's in the stool)

x Fever

x Bleeding within the rectal region

x The rectal region is painful.

x Vomiting

Also, consult your doctor If you experience any of the symptoms listed.

CONTRADICTIONS OF CHRONIC CONSTIPATION

As we mentioned chronic constipation can cause health issues in the long-term. Apart from the discomforts it may cause, it could be a cause of health problems.

1. A STRAINING OUTCOME OF CONSTIPATION HEMORRHOIDS

If you're always struggling due to constipation, it can cause swelling of the veins within your anal region. This is known as hemorrhoids. In accordance with the severity of hemorrhoids, someone with hemorrhoids could require or not undergo surgery.

2. STOOLS WITH LARGE AND HARD STROOLS Anal FISSURE

Constipated individuals typically have large and hard stool. This can make bowel movements extremely difficult. In some instances, tears in the anal region could be the result of straining. In addition to the discomfort and pain anal fissures can cause as well, it may be a risk to infections.

3. IMPACT OF HARDENED STOOL ON FECAL IMPACT

A large and hard tool could be stuck inside the intestine. Fecal impaction can require urgent treatment, particularly when there is an increase in size and obstruction within the colon.

4. STRANGERING HARD RECTAL PROLAPSE

Rectal prolapse is a condition that occurs when the rectum, or part of the rectum gets out of alignment. It can happen:

"* Partial"-As its name suggests, a portion of the rectum is pushed off the mark.

"Complete" -The whole wall of the rectum protrudes out of the anus

* Internal-The colon, or a part of the rectum can slide into the other, forming an oblique figure resembling a telescope

MYTHS and TRUTHS REGARDING CONSTIPATION

Before we go into the specifics of the different treatment options for constipation, we should learn the most popular and relevant myths and truths concerning constipation.

MYTH #1

The bowel should be moving every day. If not, it is a sign there's something wrong with your body.

THE TRUTH

In the course of daily bowel movements will vary from one

individual to the next. For example, a health person might pass stool daily, while a healthy person does it each and every day. It all depends on what is normal for the individual.

MYTH #2

I'm suffering from constipation, and all I require is fiber, nothing else.

THE TRUTH

Fiber is essential in the process of bulking up your stool to ease constipation. But, you have to realize is that constipation could be multi-factorial. That means there could be many reasons that you are having difficulty with your stool. If you have constipation that has become chronic it is best to consult your physician to get a consultation.

MYTH #3

If I consume a lot of dairy products like milk or other dairy products I'll be constipated.

THE TRUTH

Constipation can be caused by dairy products in people who are lactose intolerant or who cannot digest lactose fully. For those who are lactose-intolerant small quantities of dairy are generally acceptable. Check with your doctor to make certain.

MYTH #4

The delay in your bowel movements isn't affecting you at all.

THE TRUTH

In addition to the discomfort it causes Delaying the process of bowel elimination can cause constipation in longer term. This is due to the fact that delay could weaken the signals you feel when you have an urge to get rid of.

MYTH #5

Coffee can ease constipation.

THE TRUTH

Yes, coffee has the ability to boost the muscles of your digestive system, resulting in the bowel to move faster. However, it's diuretic due to this, it makes your stool harder, making it more difficult to eliminate.

TREATMENTS and TIPS FOR CONSTIPATION

In this section we will review the different treatment options and tips you can follow and think about to deal with constipation.

Eat a balanced and balanced diet. This is essential as the food we consume can affect our habits of elimination. If you can improve the amount of fiber you consume within your daily diet. Like what I previously mentioned in my book. Fibre plays a crucial role in boosting the size of your stool.

The general rule is that you require about 20-35 grams of fiber every day.

In the next section, I'll list the top foods that have the highest amount of fiber.

Consume light meals. It is important to eat regularly to prevent constipation. Apart from improving your metabolism, it can aid you if you are trying to shed weight.

Beware of foods that may cause constipation, such as dairy and other processed foods. Also, you should reduce the amount of food items which are rich in fat.

According to research studies Omega-3 fatty acids could aid in managing constipation. They are found in cold water fishes like tuna, salmon and Sardines.

Drink plenty of fluids If you aren't sure, or in the event that you are it is contraindicated. As per experts' advice, you need to consume at least 8 glasses of water per daily. But, the amount you drink will depend on your physical condition and activity. Also, it could be beneficial to avoid beverages with caffeine as they are known to dehydrate you.

Get active and stay away from a the sedentary life style. Regular exercise is essential not just to keep fit and healthy but also to prevent constipation.

As much as you can you can, don't delay your desire to have an bowel movement. The delay can affect and weaken the natural urge to urinate at the right time.

Ask your physician regarding laxatives. According to medical experts, laxatives are only used as a last option. Some of the most commonly used types of laxatives are : following:

* Bulk-forming - As the name implies, this class of laxatives can help to

increase the size of your stool, allowing for more comfortable stool movements. The downside to this kind of laxatives is it may cause cramping and bloating. It is important to drink plenty of fluids when you use bulk-forming laxatives.

* Lubricant-based laxatives - With this kind of laxative it aids in the process of making the stool become slippery. This is why it is more easy to get it go.

* Osmotic laxatives: This can affect the flow of fluids through the intestinal tract. Before taking this laxative, consult your doctor as it could cause electrolyte imbalances.

* Stimulant-based laxatives: This kind of laxative works on the muscles of the intestinal tract. Due to the motion it makes the stool more easily pushed out.

In some instances doctors may prescribe an enemas treatment if the patient appears to be constipated. This procedure should only be performed by professionals since it may harm the anal canal when not done correctly. If it's successful the enema will relieve constipation within two to fifteen minutes.

For those who suffer from constipation that is chronic, you might think about Biofeedback as a treatment. This is ideal for those who suffer from pelvic floor issues. If there is a problem with the pelvic area, constipation can also be an issue. The pelvic floor may not be functioning properly. It is present in obese individuals and people who are just giving birth.

According to studies that 70% of the people who underwent this treatment noticed improvements in constipation issues.

One of the most common treatments can be used is Acupressure. It is a natural healing method that involves pressure is applied at particular points of the body to treat constipation. Apart from constipation, it can also be used to fight various body ailments.

Another traditional and old-fashioned treatment is the use of herbal. In the treatment of herbal the herbs are classified into two categories:

* Bulk-forming: Some examples of this are Barley and Flaxseed

* Stimulants- Examples include Aloe and Senna

Make sure to consult an expert prior to taking any herbs to ensure that it's not contraindicated for your medical condition.

One kind of medicine which can in treating constipation, is the suppository. This kind of medicine is directly inserted into the anus. Once it is inserted, it may aid in passing your stool with ease.

A treatment for constipation that you could consider is using Probiotics. They are bacteria that aid in digestion. A few examples include Lactobacillus as well as Bifidobacteriu.

If you are pregnant do not use medications unless recommended by your physician. The best advice is to alter your diet and increase the amount of fiber you consume. Always eat a balanced and nutritious diet for your own health and the baby's too.

TOP FOODS With HIGH FIRE CONTENT, FIBER TIPS

Like what I said earlier Fiber is essential in the prevention of constipation. It is recommended to have between 20 and 35 grams of fiber into your daily diet. To assist you in selecting the right foods, here's an extensive list of foods which are rich in fiber quantity:

1. Beans
2. Whole grains
3. Rice (Brown and not white)
4. Popcorn
5. Nuts
6. Baked Potato
7. Berries
8. Bran cereals
9. Oatmeal
10. Different vegetables

Here are some easy but highly effective suggestions about fiber:

1. Try to eat whole grains as often as you can.

2. Include beans in your diet at least a few times every week, unless it is contraindicated. Beans are a great source of fiber.

3. Include fruits in your diet.

4. Eat a variety of vegetables every day.

Chapter 8: Understanding Constipation

Before we discuss how to fix this issue we should learn first why and how constipation occurs.

All of it begins with the passage of fecal matter through the small intestine into the large intestinal. During the transfer, stool is accompanied by water. But, when stool travels across the intestinal tract as it travels to the rectum of the liquid is sucked out and the stool flows down the rest of your large intestines in solids.

There are many reasons for constipation. The most common reason is a an unhealthy diet. If your diet is made up of high-fat foods high in fiber in addition, you drink little enough water often the constipation will occur. A different cause of constipation is the change in your eating habits or routine. There is nothing more disruptive to your routine than traveling. Therefore, if you frequently travel, you might suffer from constipation.

If you are also not exercising this can result in constipation. Certain antacids may cause constipation, particularly in the case of aluminum or calcium in their ingredients. Other medicines such as pain killers as well as antidepressants which contain iron can cause constipation. Patients suffering with eating disorders usually have constipation too. If you also consume excessive amounts of dairy, and you've got it, and you are constipated.

Constipation isn't really an issue with your colorectal system. It's more of a disturbance in the bowel function.

The cause of this disorder is usually caused by your diet and what you do not eat as well as the drinks you consume (and do not drink) as well as your lifestyle and even your mood. The book doesn't discuss all of factors that cause constipation since it is still recommended that you consult a medical professional in the event that you suspect the reason for your constipation is an illness that is more serious. Keep in mind that colon cancer could cause constipation too.

However, if you are aware that your problem is the result of a poor diet, an alteration in your lifestyle or something that you can address by reading our suggested solutions.

Food Remedies

Constipation is a matter that we go through in our digestive system So, the treatment must begin at the beginning. Consuming the right food can definitely help treat constipation effectively.

Fiber

Everyone is aware that food that is rich with fiber are the ideal to keep your bowels regular. A healthy diet high in fiber will not only rid constipation but also prevents the possibility of becoming constipated. Therefore, if your food is predominantly comprised of carbs and meat, consider including more fruits and vegetables or, even better to replace.

Artificial foods such as "frankenmeats" which are now being sold in supermarkets create problems due to the fact that they're not easily passed through our digestive tracts. In reality, of course it is not necessary to stay away from these types of food items. However, making sure you balance your diet with foods that are fibrous will allow you to get these processed meats much more easily. It is because fiber functions as sponges. It absorbs water and the stool softens and thus, moves throughout the system of colorectal more easily.

Plums, beans, berries or nuts, as well as potatoes (as as long as they're non-in "French fry shape") will provide more fiber to your diet.

Oil

If you're experiencing constipation, eating a healthy oil , like olive oil made from pure will ease the pain. Olive oil (or coconut oil virgin) can help keep the process "running". It will help stimulate your digestive system, ensuring that you're regularly going.

Another thing pure oil performs is as a lubricant that helps the stool. Consuming oil that is pure will aid in the passage of solid matter through your colon more easily and will keep the colon moving.

Of course, certain people will be more enthused by this method than other people. Therefore, if you're able to consume oil in its pure form, consider adding one spoonful of fresh lemon juice for every teaspoon of oil (be it coconut or olive) to aid in swallowing the mix.

You can try this remedy as you awake in the morning since it is more effective when consumed in a stomach that is empty.

Lemons

Although they were previously used in order to help make oil remedies more palatable however, lemons, on their own can also be effective in resolving for constipation. Citric acid is present in lemons that can also help to stimulate the digestive system. Therefore, if you wish to use the oil in lemon juice.

Another benefit lemons offer is the detoxification. They assist the digestive system to move and flushing waste from our bodies and flushing out the toxins that accumulate throughout the colon. Thus, you're getting rid of toxins in your body through this treatment.

Like pure oil, it's highly advised to drink the lemon water early in the morning prior to eating any other food. Another suggestion is mixing lemon juice in warm water, and then wait approximately 30 minutes to an hour after drinking the lemon water prior to eating any food item.

Molasses

It is necessary to purchase an exclusive type of molasses to use this treatment and are referred to as blackstrap Molasses. Molasses made from the same juice of sugarcane however they are made by the final boiling process (usually at least the 3rd time) They are also loaded with minerals and vitamins including magnesium which is a natural cleanser!

Make this drink just as you did with lemon water by adding blackstrap-molasses to warm water, and then drinking it at the beginning of the day. It is also possible to include blackstrap molasses in your favourite tea as an natural sweetener.

Flaxseed oil

Like previous remedies it takes some time to get used to. However, flaxseed oil can be an effective treatment for constipation. It does not just alleviate constipation, but it also makes you go to the bathroom more frequently. In fact, flaxseed oil can be a natural remedy to boost your bowel function. While many think that this isn't a great solution since it causes you to have to use the bathroom more often take a look at this: when a stool that is longer is in your colon, it ferments and turns rotten and sticks to the colon's walls. Most of the time it is this that is that people get colon cancer.

The longer the toxins are in your body and cause havoc, the more cause. Therefore, eliminating the toxins as quickly as you can is not an ideal idea. In moderation, this treatment is not likely to cause diarrhea. If you're someone who wants to eliminate the waste regularly and frequently, this treatment is suggested for you. The reason it works is that it coats the walls of your intestine and feces, but also the fecal matter. This allows the solid waste materials move through your system quicker as well as more frequently.

It is possible to add the flaxseed oil of a tablespoon into your orange juice for breakfast. It may make your morning drink look different from the norm, however in the end it will be a part of your routine for the day.

Aloe

Popular in skin and hair treatment, aloe is actually, great for digestion, as well. If you can locate aloe juice at your local grocery shop, go for it! The flavor is odd, but you'll will get familiar with it. This is an all-natural cleanser.

Aloe can also aid the digestive system in breaking down food and ensure that it can pass through your intestines more easily.

For this remedy, you can take a glass of aloe juice, or, if you own an aloe-producing plant, use two spoons of the pure gel. Mix the two and use this remedy early in the morning before you eat anything else.

More Liquids

Water assists your digestive system in every aspect, from the digestion process to the management of waste. Therefore, if you're constipated this is simply a sign that you're insufficiently drinking water. The more water you are putting into your body does more than help to keep your bowels regular, but also assists you to rid yourself of toxins too.

A suitable amount of water for an adult daily consumption is 3 Liters.

Warm water is more beneficial than tap water that is cold or cold particularly when it is mixed with other fluids that support regular bowel movements.

You can boost the flavor of your water by adding lemon, molasses as well as baking soda! Yes! It's basically the bicarbonate ingredient that does not just remove air however, it will help relieve stomach pain because of pressure. By adding a teaspoon baking soda to around 1/4 cup of hot water can help. This method also helps to re-alkalize the stomach. It neutralizes acid, which assists in allowing eliminate toxins and waste through your digestive tract easily.

Another more conventional liquid remedy for constipation is to drink prune juice. Prunes are rich in fiber, sorbitol and other nutrients that,

when combined, serve as a natural ,
powerful laxative.

Sorbitol is an organic carbohydrate
that is quickly absorbed by your
body. It helps to soften stool. Be
careful not to consume too much of
it however. A moderate amount can
help the bowel's movement, but
drinking excessive amounts can
cause it to go off the rails and you
could end up with a lot of gas, or
with a fluid-filled stool.

Massage

Before you begin going to spas or
massage centers, you need to know
how stool moves through your body.
Below, you'll be able to be able to
see how stool passes through the
large intestines.

If you now know the direction that
the stool flows throughout the colon,
it is possible that you will be able to

in a way identify the direction of abdomen massage you should perform to rid your constipation.

You can do it yourself. Start by lying on your back then take several deep breaths and locate the area the colon begins located in the right side in your abdomen's lower part. It's located that is just above your pelvic bone. We will now start the massage. Start by moving the hands around in circular motion following you colon with the left direction in which stool moves towards, which is lower left followed by upwards, left and finally downward. Ten times of this massage, increasing the pressure gradually every time you move around.

After that, apply tension to your right side in your abdomen close to the pelvic bone. maintain pressure in that area for approximately 10 seconds. After that, slowly proceed up, and repeat exactly the same thing for that new colon, but be sure to apply the same pressure that you did for the previous section. Repeat this process until you've all the pressure applied to your entire colon.

The second massage is an unidirectional movement. With the heel of your hand press again on the right side of the lower abdominal region over the pelvic bone. Then, slowly bring your entire body down with a wavy motion to ensure that your fingers land in an area beneath the pelvic bone. Then, move your hand up and make the wavy movements, in the colon's direction downwards, lower right left, lower right, downward. Again, you are able to perform this massage as often as you'd like.

It is possible to make the experience more enjoyable by using oils for massage. Essential oils are ones which are known for their ability to help digestion. Mix essential oils and an oil carrier (like coconut, olive) and then use it to aid in the massage. It is possible to use marjoram, anise, lemon as well as basil and peppermint oils. Mix around 10-15 drops of your favorite essential oil with 2 tablespoons of carrier oil.

If you're not confident in performing this massage on your own then ask someone else to do this for you. In most cases, masseuses who have experience know how to apply this technique. When you tell them about the issue they'll know what to do as well as how they can massage your to ensure that you feel free of constipation.

Eliminate Bad Habits

There are certain bad habits that we have to get rid of to rid ourselves of constipation completely. First , there is the bad habit of squeezing it. If you feel like you have to go, it's because you need to go. It is your body telling your "Hey! There's just too much waste! Eliminate it!"

The human body can only carry a couple of pounds of stool at a given time while during transit. If you keep it in, and then wait until when you next feel an need to eliminate the body, it could carry around 10 to 20 or more pounds of stool. This is a significant amount to carry around, and most of the time it's not possible to eliminate it in one sweep. What does the stool do with what remains in its place?

Fecal matter, a waste product, will certainly decay. The rotting stool is sure to damage and cause irritation to the colon and anal canal and will leave behind toxic substances inside your body.

There's a reason behind why it's called"the "call to nature". It's the body's way to eliminate things that are harmful to it. If you ignore the prompt, let alone listen to it then you're not just being in opposition to nature; you're, in actual fact inflicting harm on yourself.

Another bad habit is apathy. If you are content to sit in your home, watching TV all day and do not doing anything that you can, you will disrupt the bodily functions that need our energy. Bowel movements must be activated. While 50percent of the triggers occur through beverages and food and the rest is caused by the movement. If we engage in more activities, we add to the trigger that assists the body in bowel movements.

Another thing we often overindulge and develop into an unhealthy habit is dependence upon stimulant laxatives. They can help to stimulate stool movements, and, if you take them in the right way they can work wonders. However, long-term usage of stimulant-based laxatives can eventually make your body confused. It will stop the elimination of organic waste. It will take until you've taken the stimulant before it begins to work once more.

Therefore, in essence you'll end up drinking stimulant laxatives for the rest of your life! If your constipation is to the point that doctors prescribe stimulant laxatives, make sure you follow the instructions and only use what the doctor recommends. It is essential to make an effort to return to doing things in a natural manner.

Prevention is better than cure

If you've learned the various ways to treat constipation, the next step is to stop it from recurring. In the same way, as you've learned in previous chapters, be sure you improve the amount of fiber in your diet. If you need to alter your eating habits completely, do it. A high-fiber diet won't only aid you in achieving the bowel movements, but can also help you lose weight.

Be sure to drink sufficient water. Water mixed with other organic ingredients like baking soda lemons, and molasses can aid in keeping your bowel movements regular as well. If you are a coffee lover every morning, do not fret it's also an effective natural stimulant for the digestive tract. So, go ahead, drink your coffee. Make sure to avoid the frankenmeats, and instead incorporate more fruits into your diet. Fruit juices and fruits can help you get rid of stool faster. A diet rich in fruits and vegetables can aid in reducing your weight and help keep your regular.

Make more strides. Start with a walk. It could be a short walk for about an hour prior to bedtime or run during the day, and do floor exercise in afternoon. It doesn't matter so long as you are moving. Regular exercise helps the body move stool effortlessly in the colon.

Once you've established the routine of your bowel movements and bowel movements, attempt as hard as possible, to stick to it. Life changes such as an upcoming job or travel and stress, anxiety or depression may interfere with your routine. But, do your best to return to your routine when things calm down.

Do not be afraid to let go of yourself, even when you're away from home. A lot of people keep it in while at work, school or at the public space. But, as you've seen in previous chapters that holding it in could result in constipation. Therefore, do not hold it in. Here's an idea you might want to test out. If you are forced to go , and you're at school or in the office, you can relieve yourself in a bathroom on another floor. If your office is located on the third floor. You can go upwards to the forth floor in which no one is really aware of who you are.

Conclusion

Constipation might seem like something that is commonplace for certain. But, it could have grave health implications in the long term, especially in the case of chronic kind of constipation. Apart from discomfort, it may negatively impact your quality of life.

The book covered all the information you should be aware of about constipation. I hope you are capable of learning the essential information to apply them to your journey to be free of constipation and being completely healthy.

I hope that this book was helpful to manage and treat constipation.

It is now time to implement the lessons you learned here and begin to see positive changes , not only in your health but also in the overall living quality.

It may be difficult initially however I'm confident that you will be able to apply and implement everything I've shared with you throughout this publication.

Keep in mind that if truly want to be healthy, you must have every body system functioning normally. This applies to the digestive system.

You don't have to be suffering from constipation. If you're feeling hopeless regarding your condition, simply revisit the knowledge I've shared with readers in the book.

Also, you are healthy and free of constipation if would like to.

Thank you for your kind words and best wishes!